T0135729

Bibliografische Information der Deutschen Nationalbibliothek

Die Deutsche Nationalbibliothek verzeichnet diese Publikation in der
Deutschen Nationalbibliografie; detaillierte bibliografische Daten sind
im Internet über http://dnb.d-nb.de abrufbar.

ISBN 978-3-8325-2413-5

Logos Verlag Berlin GmbH
Comeniushof, Gubener Str. 47,
10243 Berlin
Tel.: +49 (0)30 42 85 10 90
Fax: +49 (0)30 42 85 10 92
INTERNET: http://www.logos-verlag.de

Adaptive Filtering for Noise Reduction in X-Ray Computed Tomography

Adaptive Filterung zur Rauschreduktion in der Röntgen-Computertomographie

Der Technischen Fakultät der
Universität Erlangen–Nürnberg

zur Erlangung des Grades

DOKTOR–INGENIEUR

vorgelegt von

Anja Borsdorf

Erlangen — 2009

Als Dissertation genehmigt von der
Technischen Fakultät der
Universität Erlangen-Nürnberg

Tag der Einreichung: 23. October 2009
Tag der Promotion: 21. Dezember 2009
Dekan: Prof. Dr.-Ing. Reinhard German
Berichterstatter: Prof. Dr.-Ing. Joachim Hornegger
                          Associate Prof. Frédéric Noo, PhD

Abstract

The projection data measured in computed tomography (CT) and, consequently, the slices reconstructed from these data are noisy. This thesis investigates methods for structure-preserving noise reduction in reconstructed CT datasets. The goal is to improve the signal-to-noise ratio without increasing the radiation dose or loss of spatial resolution. Due to the close relation between noise and radiation dose, this improvement at the same time opens up a possibility for dose reduction. Two different original approaches, which automatically adapt themselves to the non-stationary and non-isotropic noise in CT, were developed, implemented and evaluated.

The first part of the thesis concentrates on wavelet based noise reduction methods. They are based on the idea of using reconstructions from two disjoint subsets of projections as input to the noise reduction algorithm. Correlation analysis between the wavelet coefficients of the input images and noise estimation in the wavelet domain is used for differentiating between structures and noise. In the second part, an original approach based on noise propagation through the reconstruction algorithm is presented. A new method for estimating the local noise variance and correlation in the image from the noise estimates of the measured data is proposed. Based on the additional information about the image noise, an adaptive bilateral filter is introduced.

The proposed methods are all evaluated with respect to the obtained noise reduction rate, but also in terms of their ability to preserve structures. A contrast dependent resolution analysis is performed to estimate the dose reduction potential of the different methods. The achieved noise reduction of about 60% can lead to dose reduction rates between 40% to 80%, depending on the clinical task.

Kurzfassung

Die in der Computertomographie (CT) gemessenen Daten sind verrauscht und somit auch die daraus rekonstruierten Schichten. In dieser Arbeit werden Methoden zur strukturerhaltenden Filterung von rekonstruierten CT Datensätzen untersucht. Das Ziel ist eine Verbesserung des Signal-zu-Rausch-Verhältnisses ohne Erhöhung der Strahlendosis oder Verlust an Ortsauflösung. Aufgrund des engen Zusammenhangs zwischen Rauschen und Strahlendosis eröffnet diese Verbesserung auch die Möglichkeit zur Dosisreduktion. Zwei verschiedene originäre Ansätze, die sich automatisch an das nicht-stationäre und nicht-isotrope Rauschen in der CT anpassen wurden entwickelt, implementiert und ausgewertet.

Der erste Teil der Arbeit konzentriert sich auf Wavelet basierte Rauschreduktionsverfahren. Diese basieren auf der Idee, Rekonstruktionen von zwei disjunkten Teilmengen an Projektionen als Eingabe für den Algorithmus zu verwenden. Korrelationsanalysen zwischen den Waveletkoeffizienten der Eingangsbilder und eine Rauschabschätzumg im Waveletraum werden zur Differenzierung von Struktur und Rauschen verwendent. Im zweiten Teil der Arbeit wird ein originäres Verfahren vorgeschlagen, das auf Rauschfortpflanzung durch den Rekonstruktionsalgorithmus basiert. Eine neue Methode zur Abschätzung der lokalen Varianz und Korrelation des Rauschen im Bild aus der Rauschabschätzung der gemessenen Daten wird vorgeschlagen. Basierend auf der zusätlichen Information über das Bildrauschen wird ein adaptiver bilateraler Filter vorgestellt.

Die vorgeschlagenen Methoden werden alle bezüglich der erreichten Rauschreduktionsrate, aber auch in Hinblick auf ihre Fähigkeiten Strukturen zu erhalten untersucht. Eine kontrastabhängige Analyse der Ortsauflösung wird durchgeführt und zur Abschätzung des Dosisreduktionspotenials der verschiedenen Methoden verwendet. Die erzielte Rauschreduktion von etwa 60% kann je nach klinischer Fragestellung zu Dosiseinsparungen zwischen 40% und 80% führen.

Acknowledgment

Computed Tomography is a fascinating research field and I am glad that I had the opportunity to work as a PhD student on a cooperation project between the University Erlangen-Nuremberg and Siemens Healthcare. I would like to express my gratitude to everyone who was involved in this project for the support and for valuable discussions over the years. Especially, I would like to thank my supervisor

Prof. Dr.-Ing. Joachim Hornegger, head of the Chair of Pattern Recognition (LME) at the University Erlangen-Nuremberg, for giving me the opportunity to become a member of the medical image processing group and work in such an excellent environment and motivating atmosphere under his guidance. He was an indispensable source of knowledge and always took time to answer questions regardless if they were related to work or other issues. Furthermore, I am grateful for the support of

Prof. Dr. Frederic Noo, during my three stays at the Utah Center for Advanced Imaging Research (UCAIR) in Salt Lake City, USA. It was a great experience to work together with him and I thank him for his comments and ideas that helped me so much in improving my work. Moreover, I would like to thank my supervisor

Dr. Rainer Raupach, who is with Siemens Healthcare, for his encouragement. His ideas formed the basis of this research project and many inspiring discussions resulted in new ideas or gave me deeper inside in the exciting details of CT. Special thank, also goes to

Dr. Steffen Kappler, who invaluably supported my work and always responded to my never ending flow of physics and CT related questions.

I also thank all other members of the CT PLM-E PA devision at Siemens Healthcare, especially Karl Stierstorfer for providing the reconstruction software, Heinrich Wallschläger for valuable discussions about image quality, Herbert Bruder for providing the projection based adaptive filter, and Holger Kunze for many fruitful discussions. Furthermore, I would like to thank Markus Mayer, Eva Eibenberger, Rüdiger Bock, Marcus Prümmer, Michael Balda and all my other colleagues at the LME, Harald Köstler at the LSS and Adam Wunderlich at UCAIR for their help and inspiration.

Finally, I thank the Siemens AG and the International Max-Planck Research School for Optics and Imaging (IMPRS-OI) for the financial support of my research.

Anja Borsdorf

Contents

Chapter 1

Introduction

1.1 Motivation

Computed tomography (CT), invented by Godfrey N. Hounsfield in 1972, was the first method that allowed to generate non-overlapping axial slices of the interior of a human's body without opening it. Today, CT is associated with high efficiency in radiologic diagnostics and has become an indispensable tool in medical examinations. Unfortunately, it is also said to be a high dose application: although CT made up only about 7% of all radiologic examinations in 2005, its contribution to the overall exposure of humans in Germany to radiation in medical examinations was approximately 56% [Umwe 08]. This explains the increased interest in the development of new techniques for dose reduction in CT that was strongly noticable during the last few years. The difficulty that arises with the demand for dose reduction is its direct impact on image quality.

All physical measurements are subject to statistical uncertainty, which, in case of CT, is primarily due to the variable number of X-ray quanta measured at the detector. The resulting interference, which is known as quantum noise, is the most relevant noise source in CT. Noise introduced in the measurement of the intensities propagates through the reconstruction algorithm to the resulting CT slices. There, noise is recognizable as pixel noise. The connection between dose and image quality is clearly visible: with a decreasing radiation dose the noise increases, which makes a reliable diagnosis more difficult or even impossible. An additional problem is that X-rays passing through the human's body are attenuated differently, depending on the density and the amount of the material along the ray. Therefore, the strength of noise varies between the different measurements, which leads to inhomogeneous noise in the reconstructed slices. Especially in body regions like the shoulder or the hip, directed noise appears, pointing out the direction of strongest attenuation, for example, where the rays had to travel through densest material, e.g. bones, or largest tissue quantity.

The investigation of new approaches for dose reduction without loss of image quality is one of the major topics in CT research, today. If it was possible to reduce the noise in lower dose images while preserving all clinically relevant structures, essentially producing images that correspond to those generated with a higher dose, the problem would be solved. But how can the noise be minimized without the loss of diagnostically relevant content of the image? This is a difficult task and many methods for noise reduction lack this important property. For example, it is widely known that simple lowpass filters can be used to eliminate high frequency noise. However, it is also common knowledge that their application results in blurred edges and the destruction of small structures, meaning lower spatial resolution. Thus, always a compromise must be found between radiation dose, noise and spatial resolution.

1.2   Related Work

Different techniques for dose reduction in CT have been proposed in the recent years. In [McCo 06] X-ray beam filtration, X-ray beam collimation, automatic exposure control, peak kilovoltage optimization, improved detection system efficiency and noise reduction algorithms are listed as examples for technical mechanisms for dose reduction. Of course, since the installation of the first CT scanners until now, a lot of effort has been spent in the development of new scanner hardware to achieve high image quality at lowest possible radiation dose. The availability of faster computer systems and increased storage capability are the reason why software based approaches for reducing the radiation dose gained more and more attention. These software approaches can basically be separated into two groups: the methods that perform dose optimization during the acquisition of the projection data and the methods that try to improve the quality of the retrospectively acquired data.

One possibility for optimizing the acquisition is to use automatic exposure controls. They adjust the tube current continuously during scanning and, thus, achieve a remarkable dose reduction [Kalr 05, Gres 02, Sues 02]. Currently there are three automated exposure control techniques available: longitudinal, angular, and combined modulation [McCo 06]. Longitudinal modulation techniques adapt the tube current for different scanning positions, depending on desired image quality and attenuation of the body region being scanned. For this adaption, single localizer radiographies are commonly used. With angular modulation, the overall dose for one rotation is distributed such that those directions with stronger attenuation are acquired at a higher dose than those with lower attenuation[Kale 99, Gres 00]. This makes the noise variance more homogeneous for the different directions and consequently leads to more homogeneous noise in the images. Especially in the region of the shoulder or hip, angular modulation is utilized. The major restriction is that X-ray tubes cannot produce arbitrarily high doses. Consequently, directed noise cannot be completely avoided. Even in cases where it is possible to adapt the tube current such that noise becomes more homogeneous across the different projections, further reduction of the overall radiation dose leads to decreased image quality due to increased noise.

With the invention of CT the first publications about noise reduction based on simple lowpass filtering came up [Ruth 76, Chew 78]. The application of linear filters, however, requires a compromise between noise and resolution. Over the years, many different approaches for noise suppression in CT have been investigated. For example, iterative numerical reconstruction techniques that optimize statistical objective functions [Lang 95, Elba 03]. Iterative reconstruction techniques have the advantage that the noise statistics in the projections can directly be taken into account during the reconstruction process. The disadvantage, however, is the high computational cost of iterative methods. This is still the main reason, why they are not yet used in clinical routine. Other methods model the noise properties in the projections and seek for a smoothed estimation of the noisy data followed by filtered backprojection (FBP) [Fess 97, Li 04, La R 06]. Furthermore, several linear or nonlinear filtering methods for noise reduction in the projection data [Hsie 98, Kach 01, Demi 01] have been proposed. In the majority of the projection based methods, the filters are adapted in order to reduce noise mostly in regions of highest attenuation. Thus, the main goal of these methods is the reduction of directed noise and streak artifacts. As a result, especially in the case of nearly constant noise variance over all of the projections, these filters either do not remove any noise, or the noise reduction is accompanied by noticeable loss of image resolution.

The goal of the methods proposed here, is the structure-preserving reduction of pixel noise in reconstructed CT-images. Most publications, where structure-preserving filters are applied to the reconstructed images [Rust 02, Lu 03], however, do not account for the non-stationary and anisotropic noise characteristics in CT. The difficult noise properties after reconstruction are the main reason, why the direct application of standard edge-preserving filtering methods, like nonlinear diffusion filtering [Catt 92] or bilateral filtering [Toma 98], do not lead to convincing results. Basically, two problems are usually obtained: If the non-stationarity of noise is not considered, some image regions are strongly smoothed, while other regions show nearly no filtering effect. The other problem is that most algorithms are detecting structures based on gradient computation. If no information about the noise anisotropy is present, noise streaks are sometimes detected to be structure and no smoothing across them is performed. Comparable observations can be made for other standard approaches, in particular wavelet-domain denoising techniques, which decompose the input data into its scale-space representation. Most of these algorithms are based on the observation that information and white noise can be separated using an orthogonal basis in the wavelet domain, as described e.g. in [Hubb 97]. Thresholding methods have been introduced, which erase insignificant coefficients, but preserve those with larger values. The difficulty is to find a suitable threshold. Choosing a very high threshold may lead to visible loss of image structures. On the other hand, a very low threshold may result in insufficient noise suppression. Various techniques have been developed for improving the detection and preservation of edges and relevant image content, for example by comparing the detail coefficients at adjacent scales [Xu 94, Fagh 02]. The additive noise in CT-images, however, cannot be assumed to be white. Making matters even more complicated, noise is not stationary, violating, for example, the assumptions in [Pizu 03] for estimating the statistical distributions of coefficients representing structures or noise. Furthermore, directed noise grains are usually visible in CT images, what makes the distinction between noise and structures even more difficult. Motivated by the complicated noise conditions in CT, methods which adapt themselves to the noise in the images were developed here.

1.3 Contributions

This work investigates methods for structure-preserving noise reduction in reconstructed CT datasets based on correlation analysis. The goal is to improve the signal-to-noise ratio without increasing the radiation dose or noticeably affecting the spatial resolution. Due to the close relation between image noise and radiation dose, this improvement at the same time opens up a possibility for dose reduction. The contributions of this work can be summarized as follows: Two different original approaches for noise reduction in CT were developed, implemented and evaluated.

Wavelet Based Noise Reduction: The first approach is based on the idea of using reconstructions from two disjoint subsets of projections as input to a wavelet based noise reduction algorithm, as we first introduced in [Bors 06]. This idea was inspired by the work of Tischenko et al. [Tisc 05], where two radiography images, taken shortly after each other, are used for wavelet denoising. The algorithm was refined, such that it can be combined with different wavelet transformations and a new correlation coefficient based similarity measurement was introduced in [Bors 08c]. An alternative wavelet based filtering method was developed, which allows anisotropic filtering [Bors 07a]. In [Bors 08d] we propose a local, frequency and orientation dependent noise estimation technique for threshold determination in the wavelet domain. The weighting of noisy detail coefficients based on a combination of correlation analysis and noise estimation and the extension of the algorithm to 3-D was introduced in [Bors 07b].

Noise Propagation for Noise-Adaptive Bilateral Filtering: The second approach is based on noise propagation through the reconstruction algorithm. A new approach for computing pixelwise estimates of the noise variance in the reconstructed image was developed [Bors 08a]. In contrast to other approaches the correlations introduced to the data during the reconstruction are modeled by linear system theory and taken into account. The noise propagation approach was then extended in order to additionally give information about the local noise correlation. In [Bors 08b] we proposed a sine-/cosine-square-weighting of the noise variances in the projections and separate noise propagation in order to obtain the horizontal and vertical contribution of the noise variance for every pixel. The approach was then extended such that for each individual pixel a specific separation into two orthogonal directions can be computed [Bors 09]. The variance contribution in direction of strongest correlation and orthogonal to that can be determined for each pixel. This additional knowledge can be used for improving filtering methods, like bilateral filtering [Toma 98], by adapting it to the non-stationary and non-isotropic noise in CT.

Evaluation: In addition to the development of new noise reduction methods for CT, this work also presents some new ideas for the evaluation of non-linear filters. Clearly, the reduction of the noise variance in the image is an important quality criteria, but the influence on the spatial resolution plays an important role, too. Usually, spatial resolution is only considered at high contrast objects. If non-linear processing is performed, image resolution might change depending on the local contrast-to-noise ratio. Therefore, a contrast dependent evaluation of the spatial resolution becomes necessary, which was introduced in [Bors 08c]. Furthermore, we proposed a new figure of merit for the noise-resolution-tradeoff, we call SNR-gain [Bors 08b]. The evaluation is based on the comparison to the linear filtering, which leads to the same average spatial resolution. The new evaluation method can be used for more realistically judging the potential for dose reduction, depending on the clinical task.

1.4   Thesis Outline

The thesis is structured as follows: The work starts with two chapters, where some theoretical basics are reviewed and summarized.

- Chapter 2: A short introduction to the basic concepts of CT is presented. The reconstruction methods used throughout the rest of the thesis are reviewed. Furthermore, two major quality criteria, noise and spatial resolution are introduced.

- Chapter 3: The wavelet transformation theory is briefly reviewed and the different wavelet transformation methods used for denoising in the following chapters are described.

The main part of the thesis describes two different kinds of original noise reduction approaches for the use in CT. In both cases correlation analysis is used for obtaining information about the local noise characteristics in the reconstructed datasets. How this correlation analysis is performed, however, strongly differs between the two approaches.

The first part (Chapters 4-6) of the thesis describes wavelet based noise reduction methods that use two reconstructed CT datasets as input. The two input datasets are generated such that they show the same structure but differ with respect to image noise.

- Chapter 4: Different possibilities for the generation of the two input datasets are discussed. Two different methods for the detection of significant wavelet coefficients based on correlation analysis are described and compared in combination with three different wavelet transformation methods. Image noise and resolution are used for quantifying the image quality in the processed images.

- Chapter 5: A new approach for local, orientation and frequency dependent noise estimation in the wavelet domain is proposed. The standard deviation of noise is estimated from the difference of the two input datasets. An adaptive thresholding in the wavelet domain is performed based on the local noise estimates. The method is evaluated with respect to noise, resolution and noise homogeneity and compared to the approach presented in Chapter 4.

- Chapter 6: The combination of correlation analysis and local noise estimation for differentiating between structures and noise in the wavelet domain is described. Noise reduction algorithm can be applied either to the reconstructed 2-D slices or the 3-D volumes. The performance of the noise reduction is compared between the application in 2-D and 3-D.

The second part of the thesis describes how noise estimates in the projections can be used for analytic computation of local noise characteristics in reconstructed images and how these local noise estimates can be used for adapting standard noise reduction methods to the special image noise in CT.

- Chapter 7: A new method for analytic noise propagation through indirect fan-beam FBP reconstruction is proposed. Based on estimates of the noise variance in the projections the local image noise in the reconstructed CT image is computed. The correlations between neighboring detector channels and projections are estimated and taken into account for the propagation of the variances. The accuracy of the noise estimation is evaluated by comparing with Monte Carlo simulations.

- Chapter 8: In addition to the local noise variance the correlation of noise is analyzed. Instead of computing local covariances, a new figure of merit for the noise anisotropy is introduced. The computation of contributions to the noise variance in two orthogonal directions is described. The separation into the two directions is performed for each pixel specifically into the direction of strongest correlation and orthogonal to that. Exemplary the adaptation of a bilateral filter to the local noise characteristics is introduced and evaluated.

The last two chapters present some comparisons between the different approaches presented and finalize the work.

- Chapter 9: The wavelet based approaches and the noise-adaptive bilateral filtering are compared to each other. Visual appearance, noise and resolution and computational requirements are discussed and ideas for future research are presented.

- Chapter 10: A summary of the work and conclusions finalize the thesis.

Chapter 2

Principles of Computed Tomography

The noise reduction methods investigated in this work are specially designed for the use in CT. Therefore, this section gives an introduction to the basic concepts of computed tomography. In contrast to other imaging modalities, like traditional projection radiography, where the images are a direct result of the measurement, the images in CT first have to be computed. When we talk about images in the reminder of this thesis, we always mean the reconstructed 2-D slices or 3-D volumes. The name projection is in the reminder of this thesis used for denoting the data used for reconstruction. Different reconstruction techniques are available. However, the ones most frequently used in clinical practice are based on the filtered backprojection. The 2-D and 3-D reconstruction methods used throughout this thesis are briefly described in the following. Further, the most important quality characteristics, noise and resolution, used for quantitative evaluation are discussed. A general survey about the basic concepts of CT can be found in [Kale 00, Oppe 06]. For a deeper theoretical understanding, overviews are given in [Buzu 04, Kak 01] and [Noo 08].

2.1   Development of Computed Tomography

With the invention of CT, a new field in radiologic diagnosis opened up. The new imaging technique was the first to non-invasively acquire axial slices of the interior of a human's body. According to Buzug [Buzu 04], „the rapid development of CT" from the installation of the first scanner generation until today „has been, and still is, driven by three essential goals: Reduction of acquisition time, reduction of X-ray exposure, and, last but not least, reduction of cost". In the following some of the most important developments in CT are summarized. More details about the history of CT can be found in [Buzu 04].

The first medical CT scanners, installed in 1972, were head scanners. They had a single needle-like X-ray beam and a single detector element that was positioned at the opposite side of the measuring field. The X-ray tube and detector were simultaneously shifted along a straight line in order to take projections along equidistantly distributed parallel rays passing through the object. This acquisition of parallel-beam projections was then repeated for different projection angles. The big disadvantage of this technique was the long acquisition time, that could be drastically reduced by the development of row detectors and the start of fan-beam tomography in 1975. In fan-beam tomography, several detector elements are placed close to each other in one line such that the whole measurement field can be X-rayed at once for a certain projection angle.

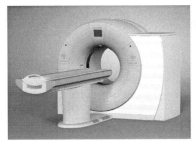
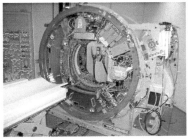

(a) Siemens Somatom Definition   (b) Siemens Somatom Definition with open gantry.

Figure 2.1: The first dual-source CT scanner - Images provided by Siemens Healthcare.

The invention of the so called slip ring in 1987 was another milestone regarding fast CT acquisition, because the continuous rotation of the tube and detector became possible. This ring in the gantry is used for the power supply of the tube and detector, but also for data transmission and communication. This development enabled the invention of helical CT (incorrectly called spiral CT) in 1989. During continuously rotating the tube and the detector around the patient, the table with the patient is moving through the gantry, leading to a helical acquisition path. Furthermore, the row detectors were extended to multi-row detectors and the so called cone-beam tomography or multi-slice CT (MSCT) was born. Comparable to the motivation for fan-beam CT, the use of a multi-row detector speeds up the data acquisition and allows to scan whole organs within few or even just one single rotation. Additionally, the reconstruction with isotropic resolution in all three spatial directions became possible. In 2005 the first dual-source CT scanner (DSCT) was introduced, where two X-ray tubes and two independent detectors with an offset of about 90 degrees can work in parallel. The motivation for DSCT was to speed up the acquisition for cardiac CT, but it also enabled the establishment of applications like dual-energy in clinical routine. An image of a modern DSCT scanner is displayed in Fig. 2.1 with closed and opened gantry.

With the development of new and improved scanning hardware, the reconstruction methods had to be advanced as well. Based on the mathematical theory on the inversion problem developed by Johann Radon already in 1917, the filtered backprojection (FBP) reconstruction was the first to allow an efficient and numerically robust implementation. Most of the methods used in the clinical practice today are still based on the filtered backprojection. With the introduction of cone-beam CT, methods for exact 3-D reconstruction came up [Kats 02, Noo 03, Denn 09, Hopp 09]. Nevertheless, approximate methods like the weighted filtered backprojection (WFBP) [Stie 04], or segmented multiple plane reconstruction (SMP) [Stie 02] are still the ones used in clinical routine for helical cone-beam CT due to their higher flexibility and lower complexity. Iterative reconstruction methods, where certain constraints can be used for handling e.g. incomplete or very noisy data, gained a lot of interest in the last few years [Kunz 07, Sunn 07]. They seem to become more and more practically relevant since parallel computing became widely available, e.g., by using modern graphics processors for general computing.

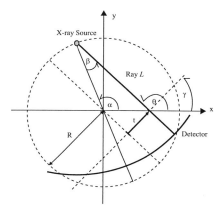

Figure 2.2: Geometry and Notation.

2.2   2-D Reconstruction

In order to understand how images of the interior of an object can be computed using measured X-ray projections, it is reasonable to first look at 2-D reconstruction methods from 1-D projections.

2.2.1   Data Acquisition Model

The basic data acquisition parameters are illustrated in Fig. 2.2. The geometry of 3rd generation CT scanners [Buzu 04] is considered here, which is currently most widely used in commercial systems. This means that the fan-beam projections are acquired with equi-angular ray spacing, and that the detector and the X-ray source rotate together around the object under investigation [Kak 01]. The X-ray source trajectory is thus a circle. The axial slice to be reconstructed lies in the x-y-plane and is in the following also called image.

It is assumed that the X-ray tube emits monoenergetic photons. The original intensity I_0 of the X-ray beam is proportional to the number of emitted photons N_0, which is viewed as a known deterministic constant. Each ray $L(\alpha, \beta)$ that passes through the object is attenuated. The intensity measured at the detector is

$$I(\alpha, \beta) = I_0 \cdot e^{-\int_{L(\alpha,\beta)} \mu(\mathbf{x})d\mathbf{x}}, \tag{2.1}$$

for a certain tube-angle α and fan-angle β. The linear attenuation coefficient of the object at position $\mathbf{x} = (x, y)^T$ is denoted as $\mu(\mathbf{x})$. The line integral in the exponential function describes the attenuation along $L(\alpha, \beta)$. It is given by:

$$P(\alpha, \beta) = -\ln\left(\frac{I(\alpha, \beta)}{I_0}\right) = \int_{L(\alpha,\beta)} \mu(\mathbf{x})d\mathbf{x}. \tag{2.2}$$

A fan-beam projection is in the following denoted as $P(\alpha, \beta)$.

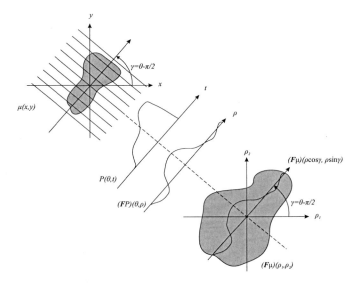

Figure 2.3: Illustration of the Fourier-Slice theorem.

Fig. 2.2 shows that $L(\alpha, \beta)$ can also be parameterized using parallel-beam coordinates θ and t. The following relations hold:

$$\theta = \alpha + \beta, \tag{2.3}$$
$$t = R \sin \beta. \tag{2.4}$$

The process of resorting acquired fan-beam projections according to Equations (2.3) and (2.4) to a set of parallel-beam projections is called rebinning. By parallel-beam projections, we refer to line integrals that are sampled uniformly in θ and t and are denoted as $P(\theta, t)$ in the following.

The linear operator $\mathcal{R}$ that maps the function $\mu(\mathbf{x})$ to its equidistantly distributed parallel-beam projections $P(\theta, t)$ is called Radon transformation:

$$P(\theta, t) = (\mathcal{R}\mu)(\gamma, t), \tag{2.5}$$

where $\gamma = \theta - \pi/2$. Goal of all reconstruction methods is to invert the Radon transformation, and thus to compute the unknown position dependent attenuation coefficients $\mu(\mathbf{x})$ from the given projections. The Fourier-Slice theorem is the theoretical basis for the filtered backprojection algorithm. It describes the connection between the Radon transformation and the two dimensional Fourier transformation of a function:

$$(\mathcal{F}P)(\theta, t) = (\mathcal{F}(\mathcal{R}\mu))(\gamma, \rho) = (\mathcal{F}\mu)(\rho \cos \gamma, \rho \sin \gamma). \tag{2.6}$$

It states that the one-dimensional Fourier transformation of a parallel-beam projection at angle θ is equivalent to the two-dimensional Fourier transformation of the function along the radial line at angle γ. A formal proof of the Fourier-Slice theorem can be found in [Buzu 04, Kak 01, Noo 08]. A schematic description is presented in Fig. 2.3. The reconstruction of CT images based on the direct application of the Fourier-Slice theorem is possible, but requires an interpolation to Cartesian coordinates in the Fourier domain in practical applications. In order to avoid this resampling in the Fourier domain, the filtered backprojection reconstruction (FBP) was developed. FBP can be directly derived from the Fourier-Slice theorem by inserting the coordinate transformation [Buzu 04, Kak 01, Noo 08]. The filtered backprojection reconstructs the value $\mu(\mathbf{x})$ according to:

$$\mu(\mathbf{x}) = \int_0^\pi \int_{-\infty}^\infty P(\theta, t) k_r(t - (x \sin\theta - y \cos\theta)) dt d\theta, \qquad (2.7)$$

where the inner integral describes a convolution (filtering) along the parallel-beam projection with the ramp filter $k_r(t)$ and the outer integral the backprojection of the filtered projections into the image plane.

2.2.2 Indirect Fan-Beam Filtered Backprojection

With the introduction of fan-beam tomography, reconstruction methods like the filtered backprojection had to be adapted to the new acquisition. The FBP reconstruction can be adjusted to directly handle the fan-beam data. Based on the insertion of equations (2.3) and (2.4) to the filtered backprojection equation (2.7), it can be derived that the projections need to be pre-weighted, the reconstruction kernel must be adapted and during backprojection a distance weighting is necessary for each pixel to be reconstructed [Buzu 04]. Alternatively, the fan-beam data can first be resorted to parallel-beam data using equations (2.3) and (2.4), followed by standard FBP reconstruction. The second approach is also called indirect fan-beam FBP or rebinning FBP. Reordering to parallel-beam projections is favored by many CT manufacturers for reasons of computational efficiency and ease in handling special scanning features such as the quarter-detector offset or redundant data.

The indirect fan-beam FBP reconstruction algorithm is now reviewed. The description is focused on discrete data. The fan-beam projections are assumed to be acquired over 360 degrees with a uniform sampling angle $\Delta\alpha$. The number of projections is even and denoted as $N_{2\pi f}$, so that $\Delta\alpha = 2\pi/N_{2\pi f}$, and the first projection is at position $\alpha = 0$. Each projection includes N_f rays with the fixed ray sampling distance being written as $\Delta\beta$. Thus, the following sampling conditions are assumed:

$$\alpha_k = (k-1)\Delta\alpha, \quad k = 1, \ldots, N_{2\pi f}, \qquad \beta_l = (l-1-(N_f-1)/2+d)\Delta\beta, \quad l = 1\ldots, N_f,$$
$$(2.8)$$

where $d = 0.25$ if a quarter-detector offset is applied and $d = 0$ otherwise. The discrete fan-beam measurements obtained at these sample locations are $P_{k,l}^{\mathrm{fan}} = P(\alpha_k, \beta_l)$.

Rebinning

The first step in the reconstruction pipeline is the resampling of the fan-beam measurements to parallel-beam data. This resampling is performed in three consecutive steps: azimuthal, complementary and radial rebinning [Buzu 04]. A schematic description can be seen in Fig. 2.4 and Fig. 2.5, with and without quarter-detector offset.

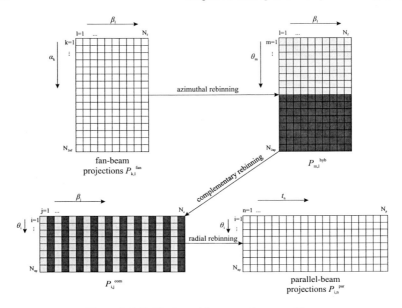

Figure 2.4: Rebinning with quarter-detector offset.

The azimuthal rebinning acts on α at fixed β to estimate hybrid projection data corresponding to samples of $P^{\text{hyb}}(\theta, \beta) = P(\theta - \beta, \beta)$. The estimation is performed at

$$\theta_m = (m-1)\Delta\theta, \quad m = 1, \ldots, N_{2\pi p}, \qquad \beta_l = (l-1-(N_f-1)/2+d)\Delta\beta, \quad l = 1 \ldots, N_f,$$
(2.9)

where $\Delta\theta = \Delta\alpha$, and the intermediate values are denoted as $P^{\text{hyb}}_{m,l} \simeq P^{\text{hyb}}(\theta_m, \beta_l)$. The relation between $P^{\text{fan}}_{k,l}$ and $P^{\text{hyb}}_{m,l}$ is

$$P^{\text{hyb}}_{m,l} = \sum_{k=1}^{N_{2\pi f}} h^{\text{azi}}(\tilde{\alpha}_{m,l} - \alpha_k) P^{\text{fan}}_{k,l},$$
(2.10)

where h^{azi} is a given, short-length interpolation kernel, and

$$\tilde{\alpha}_{m,l} = \theta_m - \beta_l.$$
(2.11)

In this relation, the values of $P^{\text{fan}}_{k,l}$ corresponding to $k < 1$ or $k > N_{2\pi f}$ are obtained using a 2π-periodical extension of the measurements. The second resampling step reorganizes the hybrid projection data onto 180 degrees using the concept of complementary rays expressed by the relation $P^{\text{hyb}}(\theta + \pi, -\beta) = P^{\text{hyb}}(\theta, \beta)$. This step requires distinguishing two cases: $d = 0.25$ (see Fig. 2.4) and $d = 0$(see Fig. 2.5). In the first case, the rays at position $\theta_m + \pi$ are interleaved with the rays at position θ_m to obtain projections with increased resolution. In the second case, two values are available for each ray and these values are

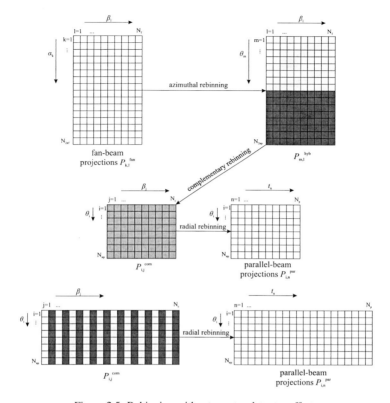

Figure 2.5: Rebinning without quarter-detector offset.

simply averaged together to get improved estimates of $P^{\mathrm{hyb}}(\theta, \beta)$. In both cases, we obtain estimates of $P^{\mathrm{com}}(\theta, \beta)$ at

$$\theta_i = (i-1)\Delta\theta, \quad i = 1, \ldots, N_{\pi p}, \qquad \beta_j = (j - (N_c - 1)/2)\Delta\beta', \quad j = 1 \ldots, N_c, \quad (2.12)$$

where $N_{\pi p} = N_{2\pi f}/2$. For $d = 0.25$, the sampling distance results in $\Delta\beta' = \Delta\beta/2$ and the number of channels $N_c = 2N_f$; otherwise, the sampling distance $\Delta\beta' = \Delta\beta$ and number of channels $N_c = N_f$ remains unchanged. The data at the end of this second step is written as $P_{i,j}^{\mathrm{com}}$. For $d = 0.25$, the complementary rebinning relation is

$$P_{i,2j}^{\mathrm{com}} = P_{i,j}^{\mathrm{hyb}}, \quad \text{and} \quad P_{i,2j-1}^{\mathrm{com}} = P_{i+N_{\pi p}, N_f+1-j}^{\mathrm{hyb}}, \tag{2.13}$$

whereas, for $d = 0$,

$$P_{i,j}^{\mathrm{com}} = \frac{1}{2}\left(P_{i,j}^{\mathrm{hyb}} + P_{i+N_{\pi p}, N_f+1-j}^{\mathrm{hyb}}\right). \tag{2.14}$$

The final resampling step acts on β at fixed θ to estimate values corresponding to samples of $P^{\mathrm{par}}(\theta, t) = P^{\mathrm{com}}(\theta - \beta, \arcsin(t/R))$. The estimation is performed at

$$\theta_i = (i-1)\Delta\theta, \quad i = 1, \ldots, N_{\pi p}, \qquad t_n = (n - 1 - (N_p - 1)/2)\Delta t, \quad n = 1 \ldots, N_p, \tag{2.15}$$

where $N_p = N_c$ and $\Delta t = R\Delta\beta'$, and the resulting values are denoted as $P^{\mathrm{par}}_{i,n} \simeq P^{\mathrm{com}}(\theta_i, \arcsin(t_n/R))$. The relation between $P^{\mathrm{par}}_{i,n}$ and $P^{\mathrm{com}}_{i,j}$ is

$$P^{\mathrm{par}}_{i,n} = \sum_{j=1}^{N_c} h^{\mathrm{rad}}(\tilde{\beta}_n - \beta_j) P^{\mathrm{com}}_{i,j}, \tag{2.16}$$

where

$$\tilde{\beta}_n = \arcsin(t_n/R). \tag{2.17}$$

In this relation, function h^{rad} is a given, short-length radial interpolation kernel.

Convolution

The next step in the reconstruction pipeline is the convolution of the parallel-beam projection data, $P^{\mathrm{par}}_{i,n}$, with an apodized version of the ramp filter, denoted $k(t)$. This convolution is applied at fixed view index and gives

$$P^{\mathrm{fil}}_{i,n} = \Delta t \sum_{s=1}^{N_p} k(t_n - t_s) P^{\mathrm{par}}_{i,s}. \tag{2.18}$$

The precise definition of the filtering kernel is

$$k(t) = \int_{-\infty}^{\infty} q(\rho) |\rho| e^{i2\pi\rho t} d\rho, \tag{2.19}$$

where $q(\rho)$ is the apodization window. In clinical practice a variety of apodization windows are available, with each selection yielding a specific compromise between noise and resolution. On the one hand, smooth kernels, commonly applied for soft-tissue imaging, suppress high frequency noise, but entail a low image resolution. On the other hand, sharp kernels yield higher resolution but to the cost of giving the reconstructed images a more noisy appearance [Buzu 04].

Backprojection

The final step in the reconstruction pipeline is the backprojection. The filtered parallel-beam projection data are backprojected to obtain an estimate of the attenuation coefficient at position $\mathbf{x}$:

$$\mu(\mathbf{x}) \simeq \Delta\theta \sum_{i=1}^{N_{\pi p}} P^{\mathrm{fil}}_i(\mathbf{x}), \tag{2.20}$$

where $P^{\mathrm{fil}}_i(\mathbf{x})$ is obtained from $P^{\mathrm{fil}}_{i,n}$ by interpolation. Specifically, the interpolation is computed as

$$P^{\mathrm{fil}}_i(\mathbf{x}) = \sum_{n=1}^{N_p} h^{\mathrm{bpj}}(x \sin \theta_i - y \cos \theta_i - t_n) P^{\mathrm{fil}}_{i,n}, \tag{2.21}$$

where h^{bpj} is a given, short-length interpolation kernel.

Hounsfield-Scaling

The reconstructed attenuation coefficients are usually normalized to Hounsfield Units (HU) according to:

$$f(\mathbf{x}) = \frac{\mu(\mathbf{x}) - \mu_w}{\mu_w} 1000\,\text{HU}, \tag{2.22}$$

with μ_w defining the attenuation coefficient of water.

Interpolation kernels

One-dimensional interpolation was involved three times in the reconstruction pipeline, twice for the rebinning step and once for the backprojection. As noted, different interpolation kernels can be used each time, if desired. The simplest and most frequently made choice is the linear interpolation kernel:

$$h(x) = \begin{cases} 1 - \frac{|x|}{\Delta x} & \text{if } |x| < \Delta x \\ 0 & \text{else} \end{cases}, \tag{2.23}$$

where Δx is the sampling distance. If linear interpolation is used, the sums in Eq. (2.10), Eq. (2.16), and Eq. (2.20) simplify to two weighted summands.

2.3   3-D Reconstruction

With the introduction of helical CT and multi-row detectors the reconstruction of isotropic 3-D volumes became possible.

2.3.1   Scanning Geometry

Two different scan modes are distinguished: sequential and helical scans. In sequential mode, the source and a multi-row detector rotate on a circular path around the object being scanned. This procedure can be repeated for certain table positions, meaning for different z-positions, as illustrated in Fig. 2.6(a). In helical mode, the tube and detector are again rotating around the patient, which is at the same time continuously moved through the scan plane. Therefore, the source moves on a helical path around the object being scanned, as illustrated in Fig. 2.6(b).

The projections now consist of several detector rows, each with a certain number of detector channels, and consequently two-dimensional projections are acquired for different source-detector positions.

2.3.2   Weighted Filtered Backprojection

As an example of a state-of-the-art 3-D reconstruction technique, the basic principles of the weighted filtered backprojection reconstruction (WFBP) [Stie 04] are shortly summarized. The WFBP is an approximate reconstruction method for helical cone-beam CT, which is closely related to the indirect fan-beam FBP method described in the previous section. Basically four main steps are necessary:

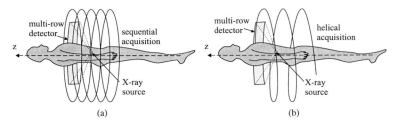

Figure 2.6: 3D-Acquisition: Sequential (a) and helical (b) scans.

- The cone-beam projections are row-wise rebinned to parallel projections. This can be performed in the same manner, as explained in Section 2.2.2.

- The parallel projections are then convolved with the reconstruction kernel $k(t)$, as described in Section 2.2.2. This is again performed for each row separately.

- In a third step the filtered projections are weighted according to the distance of the row to the center row. Weighting down outer detector rows reduces artifacts after reconstruction. Stierstorfer et al. [Stie 04] proposed a window function with a cosine-square-apodization.

- The last step is the normalized backprojection of the filtered and weighted projections. It can also be expressed as the summation over partial backprojections. This partitioning is performed, because a voxel might receive contributions from projections at one or more focus positions, depending on the position of the voxel and the table speed that is used for moving the patient through the CT.

2.4   Noise in CT

Before considering methods for noise reduction in CT data, it is important to get an overview of the origins and properties of noise in the projections and the reconstructed data.

2.4.1   Noise of Signals and Projections

The signal U measured at the detector is subject to statistical uncertainty. It can be decomposed into its noise-free expectation value $\mathcal{E}(U)$ and an error term N_U, which is zero-mean [Vest 98]:

$$U = \mathcal{E}(U) + N_U, \quad \text{with} \quad \mathcal{E}(N_U) = 0, \quad \text{and} \quad \sigma_U = \sqrt{\mathcal{E}(N_U^2)}. \tag{2.24}$$

The error term consists of two components, quantum noise N_q and electronics noise N_e:

$$N_U = N_q + N_e. \tag{2.25}$$

Both sources are independent ($\mathcal{E}(N_q N_e) = 0$) and zero-mean ($\mathcal{E}(N_q) = \mathcal{E}(N_e) = 0$), and, thus, the variances can be added

$$\sigma_U^2 = \sigma_q^2 + \sigma_e^2, \tag{2.26}$$

with $\sigma_q^2 = \mathcal{E}(N_q^2)$ and $\sigma_e^2 = \mathcal{E}(N_e^2)$. The signal is generated by the absorption of n quanta at the detector [Vest 98]:

$$\mathcal{E}(U) = c\mathcal{E}(n), \quad \text{and consequently} \quad N_q = c(n - \mathcal{E}(n)). \tag{2.27}$$

The expected number of quanta is in the following denoted as $n^* = \mathcal{E}(n)$. The physical process of generating and absorbing quanta consists of many independent small random processes and underlies Poisson statistics, which can be described by the probability distribution [Buzu 04]:

$$\mathcal{P}(\mathcal{N} = n) = \frac{(n^*)^n}{n!} e^{(-n^*)}. \tag{2.28}$$

The variance of a Poisson random variable is equivalent to its mean. Thus, quantum noise of the signal can be expressed as:

$$\sigma_q^2 = c^2 n^* = c^2 \mathcal{E}(n). \tag{2.29}$$

The intensity is proportional to the measured signal [Buzu 04] and can thus be written as:

$$I = \tilde{c}U = \tilde{c}\mathcal{E}(n) + \tilde{c}N_U. \tag{2.30}$$

The noise-free expected intensity is $\tilde{c}\mathcal{E}(n)$ and $N_I = \tilde{c}N_U$ is the error, with

$$\sigma_I^2 = \tilde{c}^2 \sigma_U^2 = \tilde{c}^2(\tilde{c}^2 \sigma_q^2 + \sigma_e^2). \tag{2.31}$$

Given the noise of the intensity, the noise in the projection can be estimated:

$$\sigma_P^2 = \text{Var}\left\{\ln(I_0) - \ln(I)\right\} \approx \text{Var}\left\{\ln(I)\right\}, \tag{2.32}$$

because I_0 can be considered to be known with negligible error [Kak 01]. The logarithm can be written as

$$\ln(I) = \ln(\mathcal{E}(I) \pm \sigma_I) = \ln\left(\mathcal{E}(I)\left(1 \pm \frac{\sigma_I}{\mathcal{E}(I)}\right)\right) = \ln(\mathcal{E}(I)) + \ln\left(1 \pm \frac{\sigma_I}{\mathcal{E}(I)}\right). \tag{2.33}$$

Based on the linear term of the series expansion [Buzu 04]

$$\ln(1 \pm x) = -\sum_{i=1}^{\infty} \frac{(\pm 1)^i x^i}{i}, \quad \text{for} \quad -1 < x < 1 \tag{2.34}$$

the variance of noise in the projection can be estimated for large $\mathcal{E}(n)$ according to:

$$\sigma_P^2 \approx \frac{\sigma_I}{\mathcal{E}(I)} = \frac{c^2 \mathcal{E}(n) + \sigma_e^2}{c^2 \mathcal{E}(n)^2} = \frac{1}{\mathcal{E}(n)} + \frac{\sigma_e^2}{c^2 \mathcal{E}(n)^2}. \tag{2.35}$$

This relation clearly shows that with decreasing number of X-ray quanta measured at the detector, noise in the projection increases. The system specific parameters c and σ_e^2 can be determined by measuring signal strength and noise at various fluxes. Especially, if the system is equipped with a bowtie-filter, each detector channel has an individual set of parameters.

2.4.2 Noise after Reconstruction

The reconstruction of the location dependent attenuation values is performed on noisy projection data. Accordingly, noise in the projections also propagates through the reconstruction algorithm to the final slices. The problem is that all the intermediate steps, like interpolations or filtering with the convolution kernel, introduce correlations to the noisy data. This makes the analytical description of noise in the reconstructed data more difficult. A detailed discussion of the propagation of noise through the indirect fan-beam FBP reconstruction, as described above, is given in Chapter 7. Here, in this section, only a very simplified description of noise in the reconstructed data is presented. All correlations are neglected and a FBP reconstruction from parallel-beam projections is considered.

The relationship between the discrete parallel-beam projection values $P_{i,n}^{par}$ and the attenuation coefficients $\mu(\mathbf{x})$ is given by:

$$\mu(\mathbf{x}) = \frac{\pi \Delta t}{N_{\pi p}} \sum_{i=1}^{N_{\pi p}} \sum_{n=1}^{N_p} k(x \cos \theta_m - y \sin \theta_m - t_n) P_{i,n}^{par}. \qquad (2.36)$$

This results in a variance of the reconstructed attenuation coefficients of

$$\sigma_\mu^2(\mathbf{x}) = \left(\frac{\pi \Delta t}{N_{\pi p}} \right)^2 \sum_{i=1}^{N_{\pi p}} \sum_{n=1}^{N_p} k^2(x \cos \theta_i - y \sin \theta_i - t_n) \sigma_P^2(\theta_i, t_n), \qquad (2.37)$$

provided that there are no correlations between different projections. The noise variance in the reconstruction can be interpreted as a filtered backprojection of the noise variances of the parallel projections, but with the squared weights. Especially for the center of a homogeneous circular disk and under the assumption that quantum noise is the dominant source of noise ($\sigma_q^2 \gg \sigma_e^2$) it can be derived that [Buzu 04]

$$\sigma_\mu^2(0,0) = \frac{\pi^2 \Delta t}{N_{\pi p} n_c} \int_{-\frac{1}{2\Delta t}}^{\frac{1}{2\Delta t}} |K(\rho)|^2 \, d\rho, \qquad (2.38)$$

where $K(\rho)$ is the frequency representation of the filter function $k(t)$. Eq. (2.38) shows that the noise in the reconstructed image depends on the filter function used for the filtered backprojection algorithm. The variance of the central pixel is proportional to the area under the squared magnitude of the filter function in frequency space. The average number of X-ray quanta of the central rays reaching the detector is denoted as n_c.

The most important properties of noise in the reconstructed datasets can already be explained based on this simplified consideration. Noise in CT reconstructions is object dependent, non-stationary and correlated. In Fig. 2.7 a noisy reconstructed CT slice, the corresponding projections and the standard deviation of noise in the projections are shown as an example. As Eq. (2.37) clearly shows, the noise variance in the image directly depends on noise in the projections. Noise in the projections is influenced by the absorption of X-rays traveling through the object. Consequently, different projections might differ with respect to their noise variance. This explains why noise depends on the object being scanned. Further, it explains, why noise differs for different positions $\mathbf{x}$ in the reconstructed image. Depending on the position the weighting of projections that contribute to the sum is varied. Thus, noise in the reconstructed image becomes non-stationary. The third property

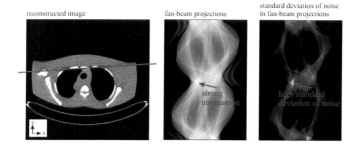

Figure 2.7: Illustration of noise in projections and reconstructed image. X-rays traveling through the object along the red line were strongly attenuated. The corresponding line integral measured at the detector for this ray is highlighted by a red arrow in the fan-beam projections and the corresponding standard deviation of noise in the fan-beam projections.

can also be explained based on Eq. (2.37). The backprojection process means that the noise variance of one projection $\sigma_P^2(\theta, t)$ influences pixels that are placed along the line $L(\theta, t)$. Altogether the variance at a certain position is gained from the sum of contributions of projections from different directions. If one of these contributing directions has a very high variance, compared to other directions, then two pixels along the line $L(\theta, t)$ are stronger correlated than pixels along another direction. This is the reason for the anisotropic noise grains visible in most CT reconstructions. Especially, for body regions, where rays have to travel through much denser or much more material for certain directions, directed noise is visible.

2.5 Spatial Resolution in CT

The discussion in the last section clearly showed that noise in CT can be influenced for example by the convolution kernel used for the filtered backprojection. When dealing with medical images, not only noise is important for judging image quality, but also the spatial resolution plays and important role. Spatial resolution tells how many line pairs per centimeter (lp/cm) can be distinguished in the reconstructed image. It thus indicates how close two neighboring lines can get to each other before they can no longer be distinguished due to the vanishing modulation of the image values, i. e., the variation of the gray values between the lines [Buzu 04]. One of the most frequently used tools for describing the resolution capability of imaging systems is the modulation transfer function (MTF). In this section, different possibilities for measuring resolution in reconstructed and processed CT datasets based on the MTF are discussed. Furthermore, the main influencing parameters to azimuthal and radial resolution and the coherence with sampling of the projection data are briefly summarized.

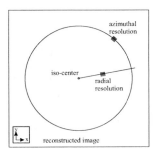
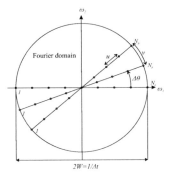

Figure 2.8: Azimuthal and radial resolution in the reconstructed image (left). Illustration of sampling points of parallel-beam projections in Fourier domain (right).

2.5.1 Azimuthal and Radial Resolution

Generally, when talking about spatial resolution in CT, azimuthal and radial resolution are distinguished [Kak 01]. Azimuthal resolution describes the resolution along a circular path with fixed distance to the iso-center. It is mainly influenced by the number of projections and the distance to the iso-center. Radial resolution describes the resolution along a straight line through the iso-center. It is mainly influenced by the number of detector channels and the convolution kernel. The difference between azimuthal and radial resolution is visualized in Fig. 2.8.

The maximum possible resolution, is limited by the sampling of the projection data. Based on Shannon's sampling theorem [Buzu 04, Kak 01], the highest spatial frequency that can be measured for each projection is limited by

$$W = 1/2\Delta t, \qquad (2.39)$$

if Δt is the sampling distance within a parallel-beam projection. The number of detector channels and the number of projections are usually chosen such that azimuthal and radial resolution are about the same. In Fig. 2.8 it can be seen how the sampling points of parallel-beam projections are located in the frequency domain. The assumption that azimuthal and radial resolution are about the same is fulfilled if

$$u = \frac{2W}{N_p} = \frac{1}{\Delta t N_p} \quad \text{and} \quad \nu = W\Delta\theta = \frac{\pi}{2\Delta t N_{\pi p}} \qquad (2.40)$$

are the same. This is fulfilled if $\frac{N_{\pi p}}{N_p} \approx \frac{\pi}{2}$ [Kak 01].

2.5.2 Measuring Resolution in Images

Resolution in the reconstructed CT image is not the same for all positions and might also vary for different directions. This makes the investigation of resolution in CT very complicated. Thus, resolution is usually only considered for the iso-center, or a position very

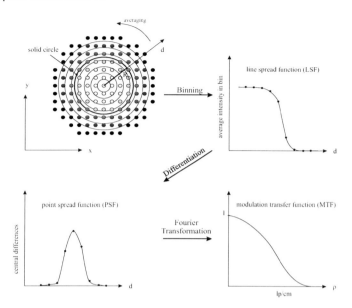

Figure 2.9: Illustration of MTF computation at the edge of a circular object.

close to the iso-center. The expression MTF in the context of spatial resolution in reconstructed CT images is rather misleading. It does not describe a linear shift-invariant system
in the system theoretical sense, but is more to be seen as a local MTF, e. g. in the iso-center.

Different techniques for measuring resolution in CT images exist. The most famous
is the so called wire method [Cunn 92]. A thin metal wire, placed close to the iso-center,
is acquired. Due to the high density a high contrast between the wire and the background
in the image is obtained. The point-spread-function (PSF) and consequently the MTF
can thus directly be computed from the neighborhood around the center of the wire. The
different radial directions are commonly averaged. If the reconstructed images with the
wire are very noisy, several noise realizations are averaged in order to increase the SNR
and get reliable MTF measurements. The problem in this work is that resolution should
be determined in images where adaptive filters were applied for noise suppression. The
detection and consequently the preservation of edges depends on the contrast-to-noise ratio
(CNR) in the image, as the different experiments in the reminder of this thesis will show.
The wire method, which is just considering high-contrast resolution, is no longer practical,
if the MTF should be determined for different CNR levels.

Another possibility for measuring the resolution in reconstructed data is, the so called
edge technique [Judy 76, Cunn 92]. The line-spread-function (LSF) is determined along a
straight edge in the image, which has a slight slope of about four degrees with respect to
the x or y-axis. The slight slope makes it possible to compute an oversampled edge profile
along the edge. This slight slope of the edge is in fact necessary for the MTF computation.

Otherwise, if the edge is perfectly aligned with the pixel grid, an arbitrary MTF might result, depending on the sampling of the edge with discrete pixels. The derivative of the edge profile gives the PSF. Its Fourier transformation finally leads to the average MTF along this line. The advantage of the edge technique is that the contrast at the edge can be varied easily, enabling a contrast dependent MTF evaluation. The critical point of this edge technique is, that the edge has a certain orientation. Consequently, resolution is evaluated for that orientation only and does not represent the average resolution of all directions. This might be a desired feature for some investigations, e. g. if the resolution should be evaluated for different directions separately. In many cases, however, the average MTF of all directions is more of interest.

Instead of computing an averaged edge profile along a straight edge, it is also possible to use e. g. a circular object [Li 07]. Basically, the MTF computation is the same as for the edge technique, except for the computation of the edge profile. The different steps needed for the computation of the average local MTF along the edge of a circular object are summarized in Fig. 2.9. The edge profile in this case is achieved by averaging the radial lines going through the center of a circle. More practically speaking, pixels within a certain distance range to the center of the circle are averaged, which is also called binning. Averaging all pixel values within the same bin leads to an averaged edge profile along the border of the circle. The critical part of this method can be seen in choosing the size of the circular object. The smaller the object the more local the image resolution is determined. If the object is too small, however, the pixel grid might be limiting the precision of the MTF computation. An additional aspect that needs to be considered is the contrast of the object compared to the noise level. If a larger object, covering a larger number of image pixels, is used, the averaging over the different directions inherently reduces the noise level in the edge profile. This might result in a smaller number of images that need to be averaged in order to get reliable MTF measurements in cases of lower contrast-to-noise ratio.

Chapter 3

Wavelets in Image Denoising

The theoretical basis for the first part of noise reduction methods, described in this thesis, is the discrete wavelet transformation (DWT). The wavelet transformation (WT) provides a tool for local frequency analysis, which is the strength compared to other frequency representations such as the Fourier transformation. In this chapter the main concepts of wavelets and wavelet transformations are reviewed, which are needed for a thorough understanding of the wavelet-based denoising algorithms. More details about wavelet theory can be found in numerous books like [Daub 92, Mall 99, Meye 93] or [Stra 96].

3.1 Introduction to the Wavelet Representation

The Fourier transformation (FT) can be used to determine the frequency content of a signal and is one of the most important tools in signal analysis. One of its disadvantages is the fact that it only provides a frequency resolution, but no spatial or time resolution. Although all frequencies ρ present in a signal can be identified with the Fourier transformation, no information about the position or time t of their presence can be given. Consequently, the Fourier transformation is only suitable for global, but not for local signal analysis.

One possibility to overcome this problem is to divide the signal into several parts, so-called windows or frames, which can then be analyzed separately. This approach leads to the *Windowed Fourier Transform* (WFT), also referred to as *Short-Time Fourier Transform* (STFT), which is defined as

$$STFT(\tau, \rho) = \int f(t)\omega^*(t - \tau)e^{-2\pi i\rho t}dt, \tag{3.1}$$

where $\omega^*(t)$ defines the complex conjugate of the window function $\omega(t)$. The window function $\omega(t)$ is shifted through the signal $f(t)$ and suppresses the signal outside the defined region of interest. This allows the computation of a local spectrum. The problem is that, due to Heisenberg's uncertainty principle, it is not possible to reach a high resolution in time and frequency simultaneously. Regarding the choice of the window function $\omega(t)$ this results in the following tradeoff [Niem 83]: the window width should be small enough to get a good time resolution and large enough to get a good frequency resolution. Another drawback of the STFT is that, once the window size has been chosen, it remains fixed for all frequencies. A more flexible signal analysis is possible with variably sized windows as used for the wavelet transformation (WT). Long time intervals are used in regions where precise low-frequency information is wanted, and shorter intervals in regions where higher frequencies are of interest. This difference between the time-frequency resolution in the STFT and the wavelet transformation is illustrated in Figure 3.1.

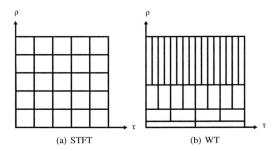

Figure 3.1: Comparison of the time-frequency resolution between short-time Fourier transformation (STFT) and wavelet transformation (WT).

3.1.1 Wavelets

Wavelets are generated from a single basis function $\psi(t)$ called mother wavelet by means of scaling and translation:

$$\psi_{s,\tau}(t) = \frac{1}{\sqrt{s}}\,\psi\left(\frac{t - \tau}{s}\right), \qquad (3.2)$$

with

$$s, \tau \in \mathbb{R}, s > 0.$$

The scaling factor s is used for expansion and compression of the wavelet. The parameter τ is responsible for the translation. For energy normalization the factor $\frac{1}{\sqrt{s}}$ is needed. The Fourier transformation $\Psi(\rho)$ of the wavelet $\psi(t)$ must satisfy the admissibility condition [Niem 83]

$$c_\psi = \int_{-\infty}^{\infty} \frac{|\Psi(\rho)|^2}{|\rho|} < \infty. \qquad (3.3)$$

This can only be fulfilled if

$$\Psi(0) = 0, \qquad (3.4)$$

which means that wavelets must have a band-pass like spectrum [Vale 04]. From equation 3.4 it follows that the mean of the wavelet in the spatial or time domain must be zero, which requires

$$\int_{-\infty}^{\infty} \psi(t)dt = 0. \qquad (3.5)$$

Therefore, it must be oscillatory, which explains the name wavelet.

3.1.2   Continuous and Dyadic Wavelet Transformation

With this definition of wavelets a local signal analysis becomes possible. The continuous wavelet transformation is defined as:

$$WT(s,\tau) = \int_{-\infty}^{\infty} f(t)\psi_{s,\tau}^*(t)dt, \tag{3.6}$$

where $\psi^*(t)$ is the complex conjugate of $\psi(t)$. The coefficients $WT(s,\tau)$ specify the similarity of the wavelet $\psi_{s,\tau}$ to the function around the position τ.

The frequency information is included in the scale s. A low scale s describes a compressed wavelet that can only detect rapidly changing details and, therefore, corresponds to high frequencies; analogously, a high scale corresponds to low frequencies. This is the reason why the wavelet transformation is referred to as a time-scale and not a time-frequency representation.

The original continuous function can be reconstructed from its wavelet coefficients by

$$f(t) = \frac{1}{c_\psi} \int_{-\infty}^{\infty} \int_{-\infty}^{\infty} WT(s,\tau)\psi_{s,\tau}(t)\frac{ds\,d\tau}{s^2}. \tag{3.7}$$

The constant c_ψ results from the admissibility equation 3.3. The CWT is shift invariant and highly redundant [Mall 99].

3.2   Discrete Wavelet Transformation

Usually, the discrete wavelet transformation (DWT) is associated with the signal expansion into a (bi-)orthogonal wavelet basis. In contrast to the highly redundant CWT there is no redundancy included in the DWT representation of a signal. The scales s_j are usually chosen as powers of two and the time sampling is proportional to the scaling

$$s_j = 2^{-j} \text{ and } \tau_k = k \cdot s_j = k \cdot 2^{-j}, \quad j,k \in \mathbb{Z} \tag{3.8}$$

leading to a dyadic sampling[1], which has also been used for illustrating the time-frequency resolution of the wavelet transformation in figure Fig. 3.1. Wavelet transformations, which use this kind of sampling are also called dyadic wavelet transformations. The DWT uses the dyadic sampling. However, it cannot be interpreted as a sampled version of the CWT. The choice of the wavelets that can be used for DWT is far more restrictive. In order to be able to represent a finite-energy signal $f(t) \in L^2(\mathbb{R})$ by a non-redundant set of wavelet coefficients, according to

$$f(t) = \sum_{j=-\infty}^{\infty} \sum_{k=-\infty}^{\infty} d_{j,k}\psi_{j,k}(t), \tag{3.9}$$

the wavelets

$$\left\{ \psi_{j,k}(t) = \frac{1}{\sqrt{|s_j|}} \, \psi\left(\frac{t - \tau_k}{s_j}\right) dt \right\}_{(j,k\in\mathbb{Z})}, \tag{3.10}$$

---

[1]Sometimes, the definition $s_j = 2^j$ is used in literature.

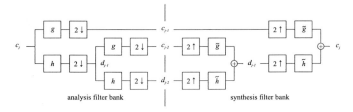

analysis filter bank   synthesis filter bank

Figure 3.2: Two-stage DWT analysis and synthesis filter bank. The wavelet coefficients after two decomposition levels of a one-dimensional DWT are highlighted in blue color.

must build a basis of $L^2(\mathbb{R})$. Then, the wavelet coefficients $d_{j,k}$ are given by the inner products of the signal $f(t)$ with the dual basis $\tilde{\psi}_{j,k}(t)$:

$$d_{j,k} = \int_{-\infty}^{\infty} f(t)\tilde{\psi}_{j,k}^*(t)dt. \tag{3.11}$$

3.3 Multiresolution Analysis

The theoretical framework for constructing (bi-)orthogonal wavelet bases and for the fast computation of the wavelet transformation is the multiresolution analysis [Mall 89]. Due to the band-pass-like spectrum of the wavelets, it can be derived that a series of dilated dyadic wavelets shifted through the signal results in a band-pass filter bank. With the constraint of $f(t)$ being band limited, its whole spectrum might be covered by infinitely many scaled versions of the wavelet. Mallat introduced the so-called scaling function $\phi_{J,k}(t)$, which covers the lowpass parts covered by infinitely many dilated wavelets up to a given J. The signal $f(t)$ can then be split into a low frequency approximation part c and its high frequency details d according to:

$$f(t) = \sum_k c_{J,k}\phi_{J,k}(t) = \sum_k c_{J-1,k}\phi_{J-1,k}(t) + \sum_k d_{J-1,k}\psi_{J-1,k}(t). \tag{3.12}$$

On the basis of the two-scale relation

$$\phi(t) = \sqrt{2}\sum_k g_k\phi(2t - k) \tag{3.13}$$

and analogous for the wavelets

$$\psi(t) = \sqrt{2}\sum_k h_k\phi(2t - k) \tag{3.14}$$

which states that a scaling or wavelet function at a given scale can be expressed in terms of translated scaling functions at the next smaller scale. It can be derived that the coefficients $c_{i,k}$ and $d_{i,k}$ can be computed by filtering with the analysis high-pass h and low-pass filter g followed by downsampling, according to:

$$c_{j,k} = \int f(t)\phi_{j,k}(t)dt = \sum_n g_{n-2k}c_{j+1,n} \tag{3.15}$$

and

$$d_{j,k} = \int f(t)\psi_{j,k}(t)dt = \sum_n h_{n-2k}c_{j+1,n}. \qquad (3.16)$$

The reconstruction can be expressed as

$$c_{j+1,k} = \sum_n \tilde{g}_{k-2n}c_{j,n} + \sum_n \tilde{h}_{k-2n}d_{j,n}, \qquad (3.17)$$

which can be interpreted as up-sampling of the detail $d_{j,k}$ and approximation coefficients $c_{j,k}$, filtering with the synthesis high-pass $\tilde{h}$ and low-pass $\tilde{g}$ filter and summation of the two parts. An example of a two-stage analysis and synthesis filter bank is shown in Fig. 3.2. As can be seen from Eq. (3.15), Eq. (3.16) and Eq. (3.17) the wavelet and scaling functions are not needed for the computation of the discrete wavelet decomposition or reconstruction. Instead the analysis and synthesis filters need to be designed carefully. For perfect reconstruction of the signal the following two conditions must hold for the z-transformations of the filters:

$$\tilde{H}(z)H(z) + \tilde{G}(z)G(z) = 0 \quad \text{(no aliassing)}, \qquad (3.18)$$
$$\tilde{H}(z)H(-z) + \tilde{G}(z)G(-z) = 2z^{-q} \quad \text{(no distortion)}, \qquad (3.19)$$

where $q \in \mathbb{Z}$ defines the system delay [Stra 96].

The above described fast algorithm is in literature usually referred to as discrete wavelet transformation (DWT). Throughout the rest of this thesis we adopt this notation. For a data array with N samples the DWT has a computational and storage complexity of $O(N)$, which is even faster than the fast Fourier Transformation (FFT), which has a complexity of $O(N \log N)$. In practical applications the approximation coefficients at the highest scale $s = 2^{-J}$ are approximated by the input data samples. If the sampling intervals are sufficiently small the approximation error of directly using the input samples as approximation coefficients is negligibly small [Wick 94].

3.4 Wavelet based Noise Reduction in Images

The introduction to the wavelet representation presented so far concentrated on one-dimensional signals. The main focus of this thesis is the noise suppression in images. Therefore, this section summarizes the main principles of the three different wavelet-transformation schemes and wavelets that are used within this thesis for noise reduction purposes.

3.4.1 Wavelet Transformations in Higher Dimensions

In addition to the separable extension of the DWT, two redundant wavelet transformations are discussed: the stationary wavelet transformation (SWT) and the algorithm á trous (ATR). In this section, the main differences between the different approaches are explained and schematic descriptions of the algorithms are presented. For the theoretical derivations the books [Mall 99, Stra 96] give detailed information.

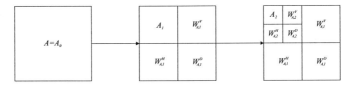

Figure 3.3: Schematic description of two decomposition levels of a 2-D-DWT. In each step the one-dimensional DWT is successively applied to the rows and the columns of the image.

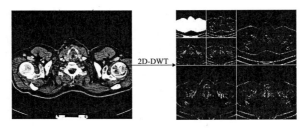

Figure 3.4: Two levels of a 2-D-DWT applied to a CT image.

DWT in Higher Dimensions

When dealing with images, the two-dimensional wavelet transformation is required. The one-dimensional transformation can be applied to the rows and columns of an image A successively, which is referred to as separable transformation [Mall 89]. The original input image is also denoted as A_0, the approximation at the highest scale or at decomposition level $l = 0$. Each step of the wavelet transformation decomposes the approximation image at level l into four two-dimensional blocks of coefficients: the lowpass filtered approximation image A_{l+1}, and three detail images $W^V_{A,l+1}$, $W^H_{A,l+1}$ and $W^D_{A,l+1}$ which include high frequency structures in the horizontal (H), vertical (V) and diagonal (D) directions. In Fig. 3.3 a schematic description of the separable two-dimensional DWT is presented. Like the 1-D case, the 2-D multiresolution wavelet decomposition can be computed iteratively from the approximation coefficients of the previous decomposition level. An example of a 2-D-DWT performed on a CT-image is shown in Fig. 3.4. The separable DWT can easily be extended to also work for more than two dimensions.

SWT - Stationary Wavelet Transformation

The computational efficiency and the constant storage complexity are key advantages of DWT. Nevertheless, the non-decimating wavelet transformation, also known as stationary wavelet transformation (SWT), has certain advantages over DWT concerning noise reduction [Coif 95, Naso 95]. Mainly, SWT works in the same way as DWT with the difference that no downsampling step is performed. In contrast to DWT, the frequency resolution is now gained by upsampling the wavelet filters $\tilde{g}$ and $\tilde{h}$ after each iteration. The analysis filter bank of the 2-D-SWT is presented in Fig. 3.5. The number of wavelet coefficients in

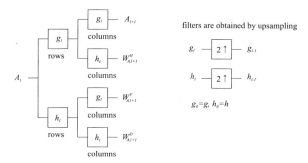

Figure 3.5: 2-D-SWT analysis filter bank. No downsampling of the coefficients is performed. Instead the frequency resolution is obtained by upsampling the filters.

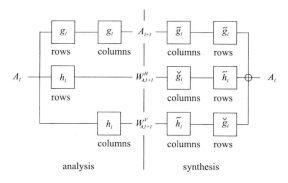

Figure 3.6: 2-D-ATR analysis and synthesis filter bank. Only highpass filtering to one direction without lowpass filtering orthogonal to that is applied in order to achieve the horizontal and vertical detail coefficients. No diagonal details are obtained. The frequency resolution is again obtained by upsampling of the filters.

all blocks (A_l, $W_{A,l}^V$, $W_{A,l}^H$ and $W_{A,l}^D$) are the same as number of pixels in the original image, independent from the decomposition level l. This leads to an overall increased storage complexity of SWT compared to DWT. At decomposition level l a redundancy factor of 2^l is included for each dimension. The reconstruction from this redundant representation is not unique. If coefficients are modified, as it is done in cases of noise reduction, an additional smoothing can be achieved by combining all possible reconstructions from non-redundant subsets. More precisely, at level l for each dimension the average of 2^l inverse 2-D-DWTs is computed.

ATR - Algorithm á Trous

A third alternative two-dimensional wavelet transformation considered in this thesis is the á-trous (ATR) algorithm as described in [Mall 92]. The analysis and synthesis filter banks are shown in Fig. 3.6. The main difference in comparison to DWT and SWT is that only two instead of three detail images are computed at each decomposition level. The approximation coefficients A_l at decomposition level l are again computed by filtering the approximation coefficients of the previous decomposition level $l-1$ with the lowpass filter in both directions. The detail coefficients are filtered with the one-dimensional highpass only in one direction respectively, resulting in two detail images $W_{A,l}^{H}$ and $W_{A,l}^{V}$. In contrast to DWT and SWT, no lowpass filtering orthogonal to the highpass filtering direction is performed. Diagonal detail coefficients are not needed for perfect reconstruction because no downsampling step is performed. For the reconstruction, however, an additional lowpass filtering with $\hat{g}_l$ orthogonal to the highpass filtering direction is necessary for the detail coefficients, in order to compensate for the missing diagonal detail coefficients [Mall 92].

3.4.2   Choice of Wavelet

Many different wavelets and wavelet families can be found in literature. In the following, a short overview of some of the most important wavelets is given, which are used within this thesis. The wavelet functions of the Haar, Db2 and CDF9/7 are shown in Fig. 3.7.

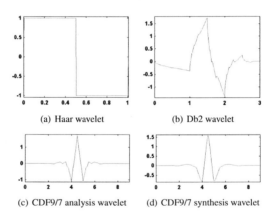

(a) Haar wavelet   (b) Db2 wavelet

(c) CDF9/7 analysis wavelet   (d) CDF9/7 synthesis wavelet

Figure 3.7: Wavelet functions of Haar, Db2 and CDF9/7, which are used for noise suppression within this thesis.

Haar Wavelet

The Haar wavelet was the first wavelet to be introduced (1909). As illustrated in Fig. 3.7(a), the Haar wavelet is discontinuous and resembles a step function. This orthogonal and symmetric wavelet is the simplest member of wavelet families such as Daubechies or Biorthogonal Spline wavelets. The analysis high-pass and low-pass filters are defined as:

$$H(z) = \sqrt{2}\left(\frac{1}{2} - \frac{1}{2}z^{-1}\right) \tag{3.20}$$

and

$$G(z) = \sqrt{2}\left(\frac{1}{2} + \frac{1}{2}z^{-1}\right). \tag{3.21}$$

$\sqrt{2}$ is needed as a normalization factor for compensating the loss of half of the components while downsampling [Stra 96]. Because of orthogonality, which is given if

$$\int \psi_{j,k}(t)\psi_{j',k'}(t)dt = \begin{cases} 1 & \text{if } j = j' \text{ and } k = k' \\ 0 & \text{else} \end{cases}, \tag{3.22}$$

the dual filters for synthesis can be computed according to:

$$\tilde{G}(z) = H(-z) \tag{3.23}$$

and

$$\tilde{H}(z) = -G(-z). \tag{3.24}$$

Daubechies Wavelets

Daubechies wavelets were the first wavelets after the Haar wavelet that were found to build an orthonormal basis in $L^2(R)$. Daubechies wavelets are compactly supported and regular. The maximum number of vanishing moments of the wavelet function N is indicated by its name DbN. The length of the filter is $2N$. In Fig. 3.7(b) the wavelet function $Db2$ is visualized. This example displays another property of Daubechies wavelets. They are not necessarily symmetric. The filter coefficients of Daubechies 2 (Db2) wavelet are given by [Getr 05]:

$$H(z) = h_1 z + h_0 + h_{-1}z^{-1} + h_{-2}z^{-2} \tag{3.25}$$

and

$$G(z) = h_{-2}z - h_{-1} + h_0 z^{-1} - h_1 z^{-2} \tag{3.26}$$

with

$$h_{-2} = \frac{1+\sqrt{3}}{4\sqrt{2}}, \quad h_{-1} = \frac{3+\sqrt{3}}{4\sqrt{2}}, \quad h_0 = \frac{3-\sqrt{3}}{4\sqrt{2}}, \quad h_1 = \frac{1-\sqrt{3}}{4\sqrt{2}}.$$

The corresponding synthesis filter can again be computed according to equation 3.23 and 3.24.

Bi-orthogonal Spline Wavelets

Spline Wavelets provide a smooth, regular and symmetric basis and have a close form representation. It is well known that symmetry and exact reconstruction are incompatible, except for the Haar wavelet, if orthogonal wavelets are used. Therefore more flexible bi-orthogonal wavelets have been introduced. Instead of one wavelet and one scaling function, as in the orthogonal case, additionally a dual wavelet $\tilde{\psi}_{j,k}(t)$ and scaling $\tilde{\phi}_{j,k}(t)$ function are defined. One $(\tilde{\psi}_{j,k}(t))$ is used in the analysis step and the other $(\psi_{j,k}(t))$ for the synthesis. How to construct bi-orthogonal spline wavelets is briefly summarized in [Getr 05]. Spline$N.\tilde{N}$ wavelets, with $m = \left\lfloor \frac{1}{2}(N + \tilde{N}) - 1 \right\rfloor$ can be generated as following:

$$H(z) = \sqrt{(2)}z^{\lceil \tilde{N}/2 \rceil}\left(\frac{1+z^{-1}}{2}\right)\sum_{n=0}^{m}\binom{m+n}{n}(-4)^{-n}\left(z - 2 + z^{-1}\right)^n, \tag{3.27}$$

$$\tilde{H}(z) = \sqrt{(2)} z^{\lfloor N/2 \rfloor} \left(\frac{1 + z^{-1}}{2} \right)^N, \tag{3.28}$$

$$G(z) = zH(-z), \quad \text{and} \quad \tilde{G}(z) = z^{-1}\tilde{H}(-z). \tag{3.29}$$

The filter coefficients for the Spline4.4 also known as Cohen-Daubechies-Fauraue(CDF9/7) wavelet are given by:

$$H(z) = h_4(z^4 + z^{-4}) + h_3(z^3 + z^{-3}) + h_2(z^2 + z^{-2}) + h_1(z + z^{-1}) + h_0 \tag{3.30}$$

and

$$G(z) = g_3(z^3 + z^{-3}) + g_2(z^2 + z^{-2}) + g_1(z + z^{-1}) + g_0 \tag{3.31}$$

with

$$
\begin{aligned}
h_4 &= 0.037828455507 & g_3 &= 0.064538882646 \\
h_3 &= -0.023849465019 & g_2 &= -0.040689417620 \\
h_2 &= -0.110624404418 & g_1 &= -0.418092273333 \\
h_1 &= 0.377402855613 & g_0 &= 0.788485616614 \\
h_0 &= 0.852698679009
\end{aligned}
$$

The wavelet functions for analysis and synthesis are displayed in Fig. 3.7(c) and Fig. 3.7(d).

Different wavelets and wavelet transformations used in the following for noise reduction in CT datasets were briefly reviewed in this chapter. Now we are ready to have a closer look on wavelet based noise reduction algorithms for the use in CT.

Chapter 4

Adaptive Wavelet based Noise Reduction Using Multiple CT Reconstructions

Recently, Tischenko et al. [Tisc 05] proposed a structure-saving noise reduction method using the correlations between two images for threshold determination in the wavelet domain. Their approach was motivated by the observation that, in contrast to the actual signal, noise is almost uncorrelated over time. Two projection radiography images, which are acquired directly one after the other, show the same information but noise between the images is uncorrelated assuming, of course, that the patient does not move. This concept of image denoising serves as a basis for the suppression of pixel noise in computed tomography images, described in this chapter, which has partially been published in [Bors 06, Bors 08c].

The main contributions in this chapter are: The generation of spatially identical input images, where noise between the two images is uncorrelated, is addressed for the case of CT. Two different similarity measurements for differentiating between structure and noise in the wavelet representation of the input images are investigated. Moreover, the use of different wavelet transformations with different properties for the noise reduction based on two input images are compared. The nonreducing á-trous algorithm (ATR), the dyadic wavelet transformation (DWT) and the stationary wavelet transformation (SWT) are compared in combination with both similarity measurements. The different approaches are evaluated with respect to reduction of pixel noise and preservation of structures. Experiments based on phantoms and on clinically-acquired data were performed. Within a human observer study the low-contrast-detectability in noisy and denoised images was compared. Finally, the proposed method is compared to a projection-based noise reduction method that is used in clinical practice.

4.1 Methodology Overview

Figure 4.1 illustrates the different steps of the noise reduction method. Instead of reconstructing just one image from the complete set of projections P, two images A and B, which only differ with respect to image noise, are generated. This can be achieved by separate reconstructions from disjoint subsets of projections. Image A is reconstructed from the set of projections P1 (e.g. from the set of projections acquired at the first detector of a DSCT) and B is reconstructed from P2 (e.g. the set of projections acquired at the second

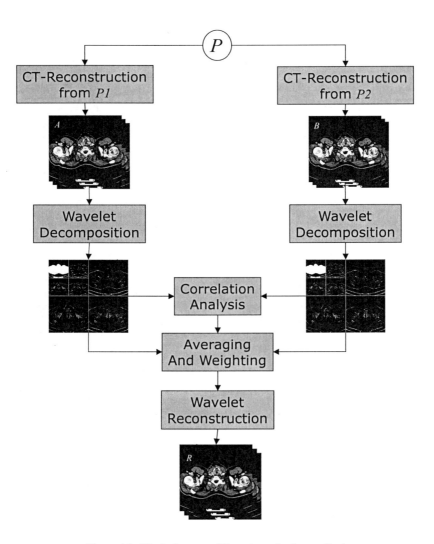

Figure 4.1: Block diagram of the noise reduction method

detector of a DSCT). The two images include the same structure information, but noise between the two images is assumed to be uncorrelated.

Both images are then decomposed into multiple frequency bands by a 2-D discrete dyadic wavelet transformation. This allows a local frequency analysis. The detail coefficients of the wavelet representations include higher frequency structure of the images together with noise in the respective frequency bands. For the reduction of high frequency noise as it is present in CT images, only decomposition levels covering the most dominant frequency bands of the noise spectrum are of interest. It is, thus, not necessary to compute the wavelet decomposition down to the coarsest scale. The number of decomposition levels that cover the noise spectrum depends on the reconstruction field of view (FOV). The smaller the FOV the smaller the pixel size and consequently the higher the frequencies at the first decomposition level. Due to the logarithmic scale of the wavelet transformation, halving the FOV, e.g., means that one more decomposition level is needed. The experiments showed, that in most cases few decomposition levels, e.g. 3 or 4, are sufficient because they cover approximately 90 percent of the frequencies of an image, if dyadic wavelet decompositions are used.

For each decomposition level a similarity image is computed based on correlation analysis between the wavelet coefficients of A and B. The goal is to distinguish between high frequency detail coefficients, which represent structure information and those which represent noise. High frequency structure that is present in both images should remain unchanged, while coefficients representing noise should be suppressed. A frequency dependent local similarity measurement can be obtained by comparing the wavelet coefficients of the input images. Two different approaches will be described. The similarity measurement can be based either on pixel regions taken from the lowpass filtered approximation images, or on the high frequency detail coefficients of the wavelet representation of the images.

Level dependent weighting images are then computed by applying a predefined weighting function to the computed similarity values. Ideally, the resulting masks include the value 1 in regions where structure has been detected and values smaller than 1 elsewhere. Next, the wavelet coefficients that correspond to the reconstruction from the complete set of projections are weighted according to the computed weighting image. If a linear reconstruction method is used, the averaged wavelet coefficients of the input images (detail- and approximation-coefficients) are equivalent to the wavelet coefficients of the image reconstructed from the complete set of projections. Otherwise, the wavelet coefficients of the image reconstructed from all projections is used for weighting. In both cases only one inverse wavelet transformation is necessary in order to get a noise suppressed output image R. This output image corresponds to the reconstruction from the complete set of projections but with improved signal-to-noise ratio (SNR).

4.2 Multiple CT-Reconstructions

The input images are generated by separate reconstructions from disjoint subsets of projections P1 ⊂ P and P2 ⊂ P, with P1 ∩ P2 = ∅, |P1| = |P2| and P = P1 ∪ P2, where |P| defines the number of samples in P and is assumed to be even. The two input datasets A and B are computed according to

$$A = \mathcal{R}^\star \{P1\} \quad \text{and} \quad B = \mathcal{R}^\star \{P2\}, \tag{4.1}$$

where $\mathcal{R}^\star$ defines the reconstruction operator, like in our case a filtered backprojection based reconstruction method. Generally, other reconstruction techniques can be used, however, the investigation of the influence of the reconstruction technique to the denoising method is beyond the scope of this work. Different reconstruction methods may also lead to special requirements for the valid sets of projections $P1$ and $P2$. However, the restrictions based on Shannon's sampling theorem are valid for all kinds of reconstructions (see [Natt 86]). In the following we assume that the sampling theorem is fulfilled for both single sets of projections.

Both separately reconstructed images can be written as a superposition of an ideal noise-free signal S and zero-mean additive noise N:

$$A = S + N_A \quad \text{and} \quad B = S + N_B, \tag{4.2}$$

with $N_A \neq N_B$, and the subscripts describing the different images. The ideal signal, respectively the statistical expectation $\mathcal{E}$, is the same for both input images $S = \mathcal{E}(A) = \mathcal{E}(B)$ and hence also for the average $M = \frac{1}{2}(A+B)$, which corresponds to the reconstruction from the complete set of projections if a linear reconstruction method is used. The noise in both images is non-stationary, and consequently the standard deviation of noise depends on the local position $\mathbf{x} = (x, y)^T$, but the standard deviations $\sigma_{N_A}(\mathbf{x})$ and $\sigma_{N_B}(\mathbf{x})$ at a given pixel position are approximately the same because in average the same number of contributing quanta can be assumed. Noise between the projections $P1$ and $P2$ is uncorrelated and accordingly noise between the separately reconstructed images is uncorrelated, too, leading to the following covariance:

$$\text{Cov}(N_A, N_B) = \sum_{\mathbf{x} \in \Omega} N_A(\mathbf{x}) N_B(\mathbf{x}) = 0, \tag{4.3}$$

with $\mathbf{x}$ defining a pixel position and Ω denoting the whole image domain.

Generally, the above scheme can also be extended to work with more than two sets of projections. The reason for restricting all the following discussions on just two input images can be found in the close relation between the standard deviation of noise σ and radiation dose [Kale 00]:

$$\sigma \propto \frac{1}{\sqrt{\text{dose}}}, \tag{4.4}$$

which holds as long as quantum statistics are the most dominant source of noise and other effects, like electronic noise, are negligible. If the set of projections should be split up into q equally sized parts the effective dose for each separately reconstructed image is divided by a factor of q. Thus, the standard deviation of noise increases by a factor of $\sqrt{q}$ in every single image. The detectability of edges based on correlation analysis depends on the contrast-to-noise level, as the experiments show. Therefore, it is reasonable to keep the number of separate reconstructions as small as possible if also low contrasts are of interest, leading to $q = 2$.

Dual-Source CT The simplest possibility for acquiring $P1$ and $P2$ is to use a dual-source CT-scanner where two X-ray tubes and two detectors work in parallel [Brud 06], as illustrated in Fig. 4.2(a). If for both tube-detector-systems, also called A- and B-system, the same scan and reconstruction parameters are used, two spatially identical images can be reconstructed directly. The image A is reconstructed from the projections $P1$ acquired at the first detector and the image B from the projections $P2$ of the second detector. Instead

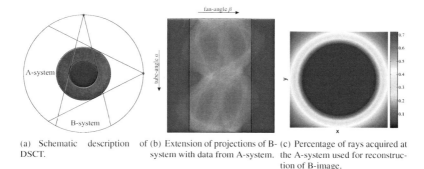

(a) Schematic description of DSCT.

(b) Extension of projections of B-system with data from A-system.

(c) Percentage of rays acquired at the A-system used for reconstruction of B-image.

Figure 4.2: Left: Schematic description of a DSCT-scanner. Middle: Illustration of padding of projections acquired at smaller second detector (colored in blue) in DSCT system with data from the larger detector (colored in red). Right: The percentage of correlated rays used for the reconstruction within a FOV of 35 cm of the B-image, where the measurement FOV is only 26 cm and the data at the outer borders is padded form the other tube-detector-system.

of simply averaging both images, they can be used as input to the noise reduction algorithm in order to further suppress noise.

In real DSCT systems the detector of the B-system might be smaller than the detector of the A-system. Therefore, the projections acquired at the B-system are extended at the outer border with data from the A-system, as explained in detail in [Brud 06]. The extensions of the projections is illustrated in Fig. 4.2(b). With this technique two images can be reconstructed at the full measurement FOV of the larger detector. Inside the FOV that is covered by both detectors independent acquisitions from the two detectors exist. Consequently, noise within these regions can be assumed to be uncorrelated between the two images. Outside this region only parts of the projections derive from independent measurements due to the padding of the projections. Therefore, noise in this outer region is no longer perfectly uncorrelated. How many independent measurements are used for the reconstruction of a certain point depends on the distance of this point to the fully covered FOV. The percentage of padded data is shown in Fig. 4.2(c) as an example.

Single-Source CT If no DSCT scanner is available, different approaches for generating two disjoint subsets are possible. For example, P1 and P2 can be acquired within two successive scans of the same body region using the same scanning parameters. This requires that the patient does not move between the two scans.

In order to avoid scanning the same object twice, another possibility is proposed for generating A and B from one single scan. Let us first consider parallel geometry and assume that noise between neighboring parallel projections is uncorrelated, which means that cross-talk at the detector is negligibly small. Then, two complete images can be reconstructed, each using only every other projection. Specifically, the A image is computed from the even and the B image from the odd numbered projections:

$$P1 = \{P_i \,|\, i \mod 2 = 0\}\,, \tag{4.5}$$
$$P2 = \{P_i \,|\, i \mod 2 = 1\}\,, \tag{4.6}$$

where the total number of projections is assumed to be even. A parallel projection acquired at the rotation angle θ_i is denoted as P_i. Under the constraint of uncorrelated parallel projections, noise between A and B is again uncorrelated as stated in equation (4.3). If a linear reconstruction method, like the filtered backprojection is used, the average of the two input images again corresponds to the reconstruction from the complete set of projections. Thus, averaging the two separately reconstructed images corresponds to the reconstruction using the complete set of projections. It has the same image resolution and the same amount of pixel noise. However, halving the number of projections might influence aliasing artifacts and resolution in A and B. With decreasing number of projections the artifact radius, within which a reconstruction free of artifacts is possible, decreases [Oppe 06]. Furthermore, azimuthal resolution is reduced away from the iso-center [Kak 01]. Usually, for CT-scanners commonly available, the number of projections is set to a fixed number that ensures a reconstruction free of artifacts within a certain FOV at a certain maximum resolution. Thus, for the application of this splitting technique, care must be taken that the number of projections for separate reconstructions is still high enough for the desired FOV in order to avoid lower correlations due to reduced resolution or artifacts in A and B. Alternatively, the scan protocol can be adapted to acquire the doubled number of projections per rotation.

A comparable splitting technique can also be applied when working with fan-beam data. Basically, two different methods for splitting of projections are possible: the fan-beam projections can be split up before or after rebinning to parallel-beam projections. If the fan-beam projections are first rebinned to parallel-beam projections and then split up into two disjoint subsets, the problem arises that noise between the two reconstructed images A and B is no longer uncorrelated, because all projections were used for the rebinning step. Therefore, it is more reasonable to split up the fan-beam projections before rebinning. The radial rebinning, however, is a non-linear operation. As a consequence the mean image $M = \frac{1}{2}(A + B)$ is no longer the reconstruction from the complete set of projections. This effect is nearly not noticeable close to the iso-center, but with increasing distance to the iso-center resolution is slightly reduced. In order to make sure, that the final result R corresponds to the image reconstructed from the complete set of projections with increased SNR, the wavelet coefficients of the image reconstructed from the complete set of projections should be weighted.

4.3 Correlation Analysis in the Wavelet Domain

The separately reconstructed images A and B are decomposed into multiple frequency bands by a discrete wavelet transformation. Here, three different wavelet transformations: á-trous wavelet transformation (ATR), discrete time wavelet transformation (DWT), and shift invariant wavelet transformation (SWT) are compared with respect to their noise reduction properties in CT based on correlation analysis.

Detail coefficients gained from the multiresolution wavelet decomposition of the input images include structure information together with noise. The goal of the correlation analysis is to estimate the probability of a detail coefficient corresponding to structure. This estimate is based on the measurement of the local frequency-dependent similarity of the input images.

Two different methods for similarity computation will be discussed. First, a correlation coefficient based measurement, comparing pixel regions from the approximation images, will be introduced. Secondly, a similarity measurement, directly based on the detail coefficients, is presented. The core idea behind both methods is similar: For all detail images of the wavelet decomposition, including horizontal, vertical (and diagonal) details, a corresponding similarity image C_l between the corresponding wavelet decompositions of the two input images A and B is computed for each level l up to the maximum decomposition level l_{max}. The higher the local similarity, the higher the probability that the coefficients at the corresponding positions include structural information that should be preserved. According to the defined weighting function, the detail coefficients are weighted with respect to their corresponding values in the similarity image. Detail coefficients representing high frequency structure information should be preserved, while noisy coefficients should be suppressed.

4.3.1 Correlation Coefficients

One popular method for measuring the similarity of noisy data is the computation of the empirical correlation coefficient, also known as *Pearson's correlation*. It is independent from both origin and scale and its value lies in the interval $[-1; 1]$, where 1 means perfect correlation, 0 no correlation and -1 perfect anticorrelation [Bron 00]. This correlation coefficient can be used in computing the local similarity between two images, by taking blocks of pixels in a defined neighborhood around each pixel in the two images and computing their empirical correlation coefficient.

This concept can be extended by comparing images of wavelet coefficients. In order to estimate the probability for each detail coefficient of the wavelet decomposition to include structural information, the computation of a similarity image at each decomposition level is proposed. The similarity image is of the same size as the detail images at that decomposition level, meaning that for each detail coefficient a corresponding similarity value is calculated.

An important point is the selection of the pixel regions used for the local correlation analysis. A very close connection between the detail coefficients and the similarity values can be obtained if the approximation coefficients of the previous decomposition level $l - 1$ are used for correlation analysis at level l, where the original image is the approximation image at level $l = 0$. For the similarity value $C_l(\mathbf{x})$ the weighted correlation coefficient is computed between the approximation coefficients A_{l-1} and B_{l-1} within the local neighborhood $\Omega_{\mathbf{x}}$ around the current position $\mathbf{x}$ according to:

$$C_l(\mathbf{x}) = \frac{\text{Cov}_{\mathbf{x}}(A_{l-1}, B_{l-1})}{\sqrt{\text{Var}_{\mathbf{x}}(A_{l-1})\text{Var}_{\mathbf{x}}(B_{l-1})}}, \tag{4.7}$$

with weighted covariance

$$\text{Cov}_{\mathbf{x}}(A, B) = \frac{1}{\bar{\eta}_{\mathbf{x}}} \sum_{\tilde{\mathbf{x}} \in \Omega_{\mathbf{x}}} \left(A(\tilde{\mathbf{x}}) - \bar{A}_{\mathbf{x}} \right) \left(B(\tilde{\mathbf{x}}) - \bar{B} \right) \eta(\tilde{\mathbf{x}}, \mathbf{x}), \tag{4.8}$$

and weighted variance

$$\text{Var}_{\mathbf{x}}(A) = \frac{1}{\bar{\eta}_{\mathbf{x}}} \sum_{\tilde{\mathbf{x}} \in \Omega_{\mathbf{x}}} \left(A(\tilde{\mathbf{x}}) - \bar{A}_{\mathbf{x}} \right)^2 \eta(\tilde{\mathbf{x}}, \mathbf{x}), \tag{4.9}$$

where $\eta(\tilde{\mathbf{x}}, \mathbf{x})$ is a weighting function. Different possible weighting functions are presented later. The mean value of A within the neighborhood $\Omega_{\mathbf{x}}$ is defined as:

$$\bar{A}_{\mathbf{x}} = \frac{1}{|\Omega_{\mathbf{x}}|} \sum_{\tilde{\mathbf{x}} \in \Omega_{\mathbf{x}}} A(\tilde{\mathbf{x}}), \tag{4.10}$$

where $|\Omega_{\mathbf{x}}|$ denotes the number of pixels in $\Omega_{\mathbf{x}}$. For normalization the mean value of η in $\Omega_{\mathbf{x}}$ is needed:

$$\bar{\eta}_{\mathbf{x}} = \frac{1}{|\Omega_{\mathbf{x}}|} \sum_{\tilde{\mathbf{x}} \in \Omega_{\mathbf{x}}} \eta(\tilde{\mathbf{x}}, \mathbf{x}). \tag{4.11}$$

The function $\eta(\tilde{\mathbf{x}}, \mathbf{x})$ is, on the one hand, used for defining the local neighborhood $\Omega_{\mathbf{x}}$ within the image domain Ω around the pixel $\mathbf{x}$ that contributes to the local correlation analysis:

$$\Omega_{\mathbf{x}} = \{\tilde{\mathbf{x}} \,|\, \tilde{\mathbf{x}} \in \Omega \wedge \eta(\tilde{\mathbf{x}}, \mathbf{x}) > \epsilon \}, \tag{4.12}$$

where $\epsilon \geq 0$ is a small number. On the other hand, different locally dependent weights can be used, such that some pixels are considered more than others, e. g. the intensities at positions $\tilde{\mathbf{x}}$ very close to $\mathbf{x}$ can be weighted stronger than those farther away.

With this definition it is possible to directly use those approximation coefficients for the correlation analysis, which mainly influenced the detail coefficient at position $\mathbf{x}$ at level l through the computation of the wavelet transformation. The multiresolution wavelet decomposition is computed iteratively. Thus, the detail coefficients at level l are the result of the convolution of the approximation image at level $l - 1$ with the respective analysis lowpass g_l and highpass h_l filters. During the computation of the inverse wavelet transformation, the approximation image at level $l - 1$ is reconstructed by summing up the approximation and detail coefficients at level l filtered with the synthesis filters $\tilde{g}_l$ and $\tilde{h}_l$. The wavelets used here, all lead to spatially limited filters. Consequently, a detail coefficient at a certain position is influenced by a certain number of pixels from the approximation image and has influence to a defined region of pixels in the approximation image due to the reconstruction. These relations are considered for the definition of η. For this purpose the function ξ is defined first:

$$\xi(\mathbf{x}) = |\tilde{g}_l(x)\tilde{h}_l(y) * g_l(x)h_l(y)| + |\tilde{h}_l(x)\tilde{g}_l(y) * h_l(x)g_l(y)| + |\tilde{g}_l(x)\tilde{g}_l(y) * g_l(x)g_l(y)|, \tag{4.13}$$

which is then shifted such that is symmetric to the origin. The function η can then be defined such that exactly those coefficients of the approximation image of the level $l-1$ that

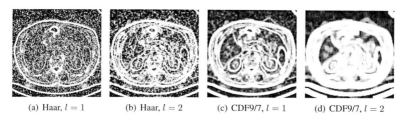

(a) Haar, $l = 1$ (b) Haar, $l = 2$ (c) CDF9/7, $l = 1$ (d) CDF9/7, $l = 2$

Figure 4.3: Similarity measurement based on correlation coefficients using the Haar and CDF9/7 wavelet for the first two decomposition levels of DWT.

have influenced a certain detail coefficient and that are influenced by that detail coefficient through the inverse transformation are considered for the correlation analysis:

$$\eta^{\text{rec}}(\tilde{\mathbf{x}}, \mathbf{x}) = \begin{cases} 1 & \text{if } \xi(\mathbf{x} - \tilde{\mathbf{x}}) > 0 \\ 0 & \text{otherwise} \end{cases} \quad (4.14)$$

With this definition of η the region around the position $\mathbf{x}$ takes into account all the pixels from the approximation image that are directly connected to the certain pixel at $\mathbf{x}$ through the wavelet analysis and syntheses steps. All coefficients within the so defined region are equally weighted for the correlation analysis. The maximum number of coefficients within this region amounts to $(2n)^2$, where n is the length of the wavelet filters, if $\epsilon = 0$. Without loss of generality the filters here are assumed to be of equal and even length.

Another possibility is to use the weights of ξ for computing a weighted correlation coefficient with

$$\eta^{\text{fil}}(\tilde{\mathbf{x}}, \mathbf{x}) = \xi(\mathbf{x} - \tilde{\mathbf{x}}). \quad (4.15)$$

This weighting directly takes into account the weights of the analysis and synthesis filters. Usually, the wavelet filters are close to 0 at the outer borders. These coefficients have a lower impact on the correlation value if η^{fil} is used.

The weighting function on the other hand can also be a Gaussian function that decays with increasing Euclidean distance of $\mathbf{x}$ and $\tilde{\mathbf{x}}$:

$$\eta^{\text{gau}}(\tilde{\mathbf{x}}, \mathbf{x}) = \frac{1}{\sigma_g \sqrt{2\pi}} e^{-\frac{\|\mathbf{x} - \tilde{\mathbf{x}}\|_2^2}{2\sigma_g^2}}. \quad (4.16)$$

If η^{gau} is used, $\epsilon > 0$ should be used in order to restrict the region for correlation analysis to a certain well defined neighborhood, because the Gaussian function only asymptotically goes to 0 with increasing distance of $\mathbf{x}$ and $\tilde{\mathbf{x}}$.

4.3.2 Gradient Approximation

The core idea of a gradient-based similarity measurement is to exploit the fact that the horizontal and vertical detail coefficients W_l^{V} and W_l^{H} can be interpreted as approximations of the partial derivatives of the approximation image at level $l - 1$. In the case of the Haar wavelet, for example, the application of the highpass filter is equivalent to the computation of finite differences. Coefficients in W_l^{V} show high values at positions where

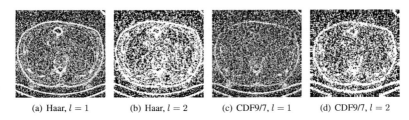

(a) Haar, $l = 1$ (b) Haar, $l = 2$ (c) CDF9/7, $l = 1$ (d) CDF9/7, $l = 2$

Figure 4.4: Similarity measurement based on approximated gradients using the Haar and CDF9/7 wavelet for the first two decomposition levels of DWT.

high frequencies in the x-direction are present, while coefficients in W_l^H have high values where high frequencies in the y-direction can be found. The detail coefficients in horizontal and vertical direction of both decompositions are considered as approximations of the gradient vectors. The similarity can then be measured by computing the angle between the corresponding approximated gradient vectors. The goal is to obtain a similarity value in the range $[-1; 1]$, similar to the correlation computations of eq. 4.7. Therefore, the cosine of the angle is computed:

$$C_l(\mathbf{x}) = \frac{W_{A,l}^V(\mathbf{x})W_{B,l}^V(\mathbf{x}) + W_{A,l}^H(\mathbf{x})W_{B,l}^H(\mathbf{x})}{\sqrt{\left(W_{A,l}^V(\mathbf{x})\right)^2 + \left(W_{A,l}^H(\mathbf{x})\right)^2}\sqrt{\left(W_{B,l}^V(\mathbf{x})\right)^2 + \left(W_{B,l}^H(\mathbf{x})\right)^2}}, \tag{4.17}$$

where the index A refers to the first and B to the second input image.

This kind of similarity measurement has also been used by Tischenko [Tisc 05] in combination with the á-trous wavelet decomposition. As already explained in Section 3.4.1, only horizontal and vertical detail coefficients are computed in the case of the á-trous algorithm. However, the additional lowpass filtering orthogonal to the highpass filtering direction in the case of DWT and SWT is advantageous with respect to edge detection. The only problem is that the gradient approximation, as introduced so far, in the case of DWT and SWT, can sometimes lead to visible artifacts. Fig. 4.5(a) and the difference images in Fig. 4.5(b) show four example regions where this problem can be seen using the Haar wavelet.

Noticeably, artifacts predominantly emerge where diagonal structures appear in the image, and their shape, in general further justifies the assumption that diagonal coefficients are falsely weighted down. The different sizes of the artifacts are due to errors at different decomposition levels. Suppression of correlated diagonal structures at a coarser level influences a larger region in the reconstructed image. The reason for these types of artifacts is that diagonal patterns exist, which lead to vanishing detail coefficients in horizontal and vertical direction. If the L2-norm of one of the approximated gradient vectors is too small or even zero, no reliable information about the existence of correlated diagonal structures can be obtained from Equation (4.17).

The simplest solution for eliminating such artifacts is to weight only the detail coefficients W_l^V and W_l^H based on the similarity measurement C_l and leave the diagonal coefficients W_l^D unchanged. As expected, this avoids artifacts in the resulting images, but, unfortunately, noise included in the diagonal coefficients is not removed, leading to a

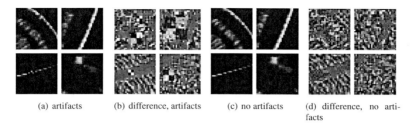

(a) artifacts   (b) difference, artifacts   (c) no artifacts   (d) difference, no artifacts

Figure 4.5: Artifacts due to weighting down correlated diagonal coefficients with the gradient approximation method - (a) four detailed regions showing artifacts, (b) difference between noise suppressed and original image regions showing artifacts, (c) same image regions without visible artifacts, (d) differences without visible artifact after appropriate weighting of diagonal detail coefficients.

lower signal-to-noise ratio in the denoised images. Equation (4.17) shows that the similarity value is computed only from W_l^V and W_l^H. The diagonal coefficients do not influence C_l. In order to avoid artifacts while still reducing noise in the diagonal coefficients, the detail coefficients W_l^V and W_l^H are weighted depending on the similarity measurement computed from Equation (4.17). The diagonal detail coefficients are then treated separately. The new weighting function for the diagonal coefficients is based on the following correlation analysis between $W_{A,l}^D$ and $W_{B,l}^D$:

$$C_l^{HH}(\mathbf{x}) = \frac{2W_{A,l}^D(\mathbf{x})W_{B,l}^D(\mathbf{x})}{\left(W_{A,l}^D(\mathbf{x})\right)^2 + \left(W_{B,l}^D(\mathbf{x})\right)^2}. \qquad (4.18)$$

Using this extension for a separate weighting of diagonal coefficients, denoising results without visible artifacts are obtained(see Figure 4.5(d)).

Note that, equations (4.7, 4.17, 4.18) are only defined for non-zero denominators. However, in all three cases it can be assumed that no relevant high frequency details are present if the denominator is 0 and, therefore, the similarity value is set to 0.

4.3.3 Weighting of Coefficients

The result of the correlation analysis is a set of similarity images C_l with values in the range $[-1; 1]$. The closer the values are to 1, the higher the probability that structure is present. Consequently, the detail coefficient at the corresponding position should remain. The lower the similarity value, the higher the probability that the corresponding detail coefficient includes only noise and, therefore, should be suppressed. We now have to define a weighting function $w(C_l(\mathbf{x}))$, that maps the values in the similarity images to weights in the range $[0; 1]$. If a linear reconstruction method is used, the weights are pointwise multiplied to the averaged detail coefficients of the two input images:

$$W_{R,l}(\mathbf{x}) = \frac{1}{2}\left(W_{A,l}(\mathbf{x}) + W_{B,l}(\mathbf{x})\right) \cdot w(C_l(\mathbf{x})), \quad \forall l \in [1, l_{max}], \qquad (4.19)$$

obtaining the detail coefficients $W_{R,l}$ of the output image R. The approximation images of the two input images are only averaged:

$$R_{l_{\max}}(\mathbf{x}) = \frac{1}{2}\left(A_{l_{\max}}(\mathbf{x}) + B_{l_{\max}}(\mathbf{x})\right). \tag{4.20}$$

Otherwise, instead of averaging the wavelet coefficients of A and B, the wavelet coefficients of the image reconstructed from the complete set of projections are used.

The simplest possible method for a weighting function is to use a thresholding approach. If the similarity value C_l at a certain position is above a defined value the weight is 1 and the detail coefficient is kept unchanged, otherwise it is set to zero. Generally, the use of continuous weighting functions, where no hard decision about keeping or discarding coefficients is required, leads to better results. In principle one can use any continuous, monotonically decreasing function with range $[0;1]$, such that 1 maps to similarity values close to 1. We use the weighting function

$$w(C_l(\mathbf{x})) = \left(\frac{1}{2}\left(C_l(\mathbf{x}) + 1\right)\right)^p \in [0,1], \tag{4.21}$$

which has a simple geometric interpretation. In the case of the gradient approximation method, the similarity values correspond to the cosine of the angle between the gradient vectors. In the case of the correlation coefficients, the similarity value can be interpreted as the cosine of the angle between the n-dimensional vectors of pixel values taken from pixel regions of A_l and B_l (both zero-mean normalized within the pixel region). Here, n is the number of pixels in $\Omega_{\mathbf{x}}$. Eq. (4.21), therefore, leads to a simple cosine weighting, shifted and scaled to the interval $[0;1]$, where the power $p \in \mathbb{R}$ controls the amount of noise suppression. With increasing p values the function goes to 0 more rapidly, but still leads to weights close to 1 for similarity values close to 1.

All different steps of the noise reduction method, as shown in Fig. 4.1, are now described: the generation of the input images A and B, different possibilities for wavelet decomposition were pointed out, a new similarity measure between the wavelet coefficients of the input images based on correlation analysis, an artifact-free extension to gradient-based approximations of correlation analysis, and a technique for weighting the averaged details. The final step is to reconstruct the noise suppressed result image R by an inverse wavelet transformation from the averaged and weighted wavelet coefficients.

4.4 Experimental Evaluation

For the evaluation of the described methods, experiments both on phantom and clinically-acquired data were performed.

4.4.1 Noise and Resolution

In order to evaluate the performance of the noise reduction methods, mainly two aspects are of interest: the amount of noise reduction and, even more importantly, the preservation of anatomical structures.

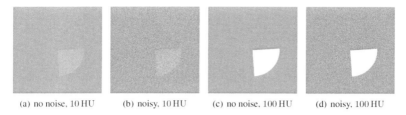

(a) no noise, 10 HU   (b) noisy, 10 HU   (c) no noise, 100 HU   (d) noisy, 100 HU

Figure 4.6: Reconstructed simulated phantom images using S80 kernel.

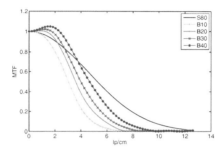

Figure 4.7: MTFs of different reconstruction kernels.

Phantom

For the experiments reconstructions from a simulated cylindrical water phantom ($r = 15\,\mathrm{cm}$), with an embedded, quartered cylinder ($r = 6\,\mathrm{cm}$) were used. The contrast of the embedded object in comparison to water varied between 10 and 100 HU. The dose of radiation ($100\,\mathrm{mAs}/1160$ projections) was kept constant for all simulations, leading to a nearly constant pixel noise in the homogeneous area of the water cylinder. All simulations were performed with the *DRASIM* software package provided by Siemens Healthcare [Stie 02]. The advantage of simulations is that in addition to noisy projections (with Poisson distributed noise according to quantum statistics), ideal, noise-free data can also be produced and we have ground truth data. All slices were of size 512×512 and were reconstructed within a field of view of $20\,\mathrm{cm}$ using: a) a sharp Shepp-Logan (S80) filtering kernel, leading to a pixel noise of approximately $7.6\,\mathrm{HU}$ in the homogeneous image region in the reconstruction from the complete set of projections; and b) a smoother body kernel (B40), leading to a pixel noise of approximately $5.2\,\mathrm{HU}$. For noise-resolution measurements some additional typical body kernels were utilized. The MTFs of all used kernels are shown in Fig. 4.7. The standard deviation of noise in the separately reconstructed images is about $\sqrt{2}$ times higher (see Eq. (4.4)). Two examples (10 and 100 HU) are shown in Fig. 4.6. For both contrast levels, one of the noisy input images and the corresponding noise-free images are shown.

MTF Computation

First, the capability of the noise reduction algorithm to detect edges of a given contrast in the presence of noise was investigated. The local modulation transfer function (MTF), measured at an edge, for detecting changes due to the weighting of wavelet coefficients during noise suppression. As described in Section 2.5.2, it is possible to determine the MTF directly from the edge in an image. For this purpose, a fixed region of 20×125 pixels around an edge (with a slope of approx. 4 degrees) was selected. Reliable measurements of the MTF from this edge technique can only be achieved if the contrast of the edge is much higher than the pixel noise in the images [Cunn 92]. Ideally, one should measure MTF on noise-free images. However, measuring the quality of edge preservation based on the contrast of the edge in the presence of noise is of interest here.

The impact of the weighting in the wavelet domain during noise suppression to the ideal signal should be measured. For that purpose, in addition to the noisy input images, which are a superposition of ideal signal and noise, an ideal image, free of noise, is simulated and reconstructed. The noise-free image is also decomposed into its wavelet coefficients. The weighting image is generated from the similarity computations from the wavelet coefficients of the noisy input images, as explained in the previous section. In order to measure the impact of the weighting to the ideal signal, the detail coefficients of the noise-free image were point-wise multiplied with the computed weights. The image gained from the inverse wavelet transformation of the weighted coefficients of the noise-free image shows the influence of the noise suppression method on structures directly. Edges, which were detected as correlated structures, are preserved. If an edge was not detected correctly, the edge gets blurred, which influences the MTF.

Evaluation of Edge-Preservation

In the first test, the influence of the noise suppression method to the MTF was evaluated with regard to the contrast of the edge. Phantom images were used, as described above, reconstructed with the S80 kernel, with varying contrasts at the edge (10, 20, 40, 60, 80 and 100 HU). The noise suppression method was performed for the first three decomposition levels using a CDF9/7 wavelet. In all cases a continuous weighting function was utilized, as presented in Eq. (4.21). The MTF was computed for the modified noise-free images and compared to the MTF of the ideal image, without modifications, reconstructed from the complete set of projections. The results of this test are illustrated in Fig. 4.8, allowing a comparison of the different wavelet transformation methods and the *Corr* and *Grad* approaches for similarity computation. Ideally, the noise reduction methods do not influence the MTF in any respect. Specifically, the edge is not blurred. If the corresponding MTF falls below the original ideal curve, this indicates that the edge is smoothed. Alternatively, the MTF raises if some frequencies are amplified. As seen in Fig. 4.8 the *Corr* method leads to better edge detection in comparison to the *Grad* approach for all cases.

This can be explained by the better statistical properties of the similarity evaluation based on correlation coefficients between pixel regions. More values are included in the correlation computations and, therefore, the results are more reliable. As expected, the approximated gradients are more sensitive to noise. For all methods it can be seen that decreasing edge contrast results in decreasing MTF. This clearly shows that decreasing CNR lowers the probability that the edge can be perfectly detected. However, one can see

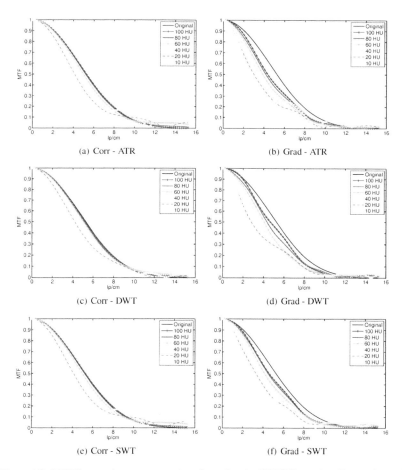

Figure 4.8: MTF for varying contrast at the edge using the CDF9/7 wavelet. Comparison of correlation coefficient approach (Corr) and gradient approximation (Grad) in combination with different wavelet transformations.

that with increasing contrast, the MTF gets closer to the ideal MTF. In the case of the *Corr* method the difference to the ideal MTF, even for a contrast of 60 HU, is very small. The *Grad* approach, in contrast, does not reach the ideal MTF even for an edge contrast of 100 HU. One can also observe that the performances for the three different wavelet computation methods are quite similar. The two nonreducing transformations give slightly better results in case of the *Corr* method, at least for higher contrasts. In combination with the *Grad* method, ART and SWT slightly outperform DWT. The redundant information included in nonreducing wavelet transformations, such as ATR and SWT, leads to an additional smoothing. The similarity is evaluated for all coefficients. The reconstruction from the weighted redundant data, therefore, leads to smoothed results. On the other hand, the additional lowpass filtering orthogonal to the highpass filtering direction, in the case of DWT and SWT, improves the edge detection results. Altogether, this explains why SWT, which combines both positive aspects, gives best results.

An even better comparison of the results can be obtained regarding the ρ_{50} values. This is the resolution for which the MTF reaches a value of 0.5. In Fig. 4.9, ρ_{50} is plotted against the contrast of the edge for the different methods. This time, three different wavelets (Haar, Db2 and CDF9/7) are compared. Two different convolution kernels (S80 and B40) were used for image reconstruction (see MTFs in Fig. 4.7). Using a smoothing kernel changes the image resolution, as well as the noise characteristics. From Fig. 4.9 it can be seen that the resolution in the original image using the B40 kernel is lower than for the S80 kernel. In addition to that, the noise level is also lower (see next paragraph on noise evaluation) using the B40 kernel. Due to the better signal-to-noise-level in the input images the edges can be better preserved when using B40. All other effects are similar for both cases. First of all, it can be seen that the clear differences between the *Corr* and *Grad* methods decrease when using the Db2 and the Haar wavelet. The results of the *Grad* approach get better with decreasing length of the wavelet filters. More specifically, the better the highpass filter of the wavelet is in spatially localizing edges, the better the results of the *Grad* method. For the Haar wavelet, we can see that ρ_{50} even exceeds the ρ_{50} value of the ideal image. This can be attributed to the discontinuity of the wavelet, which can lead to rising higher frequencies during noise suppression.

Evaluation of Noise Reduction

The same phantom images were used for evaluating the noise reduction rate. The use of simulations has the advantage that an ideal, noise-free image is available. Therefore, noise in the images can be clearly separated from the information by computing the differences from the ideal image. The effect of the noise reduction algorithm can be evaluated by comparing the standard deviation of noise in the noise-suppressed images to that in the average of the input images. Two different regions, each 100×100 pixels, were used and the standard deviation of the pixel values in the difference images were evaluated. The first region was taken from a homogeneous area. Here, the achievable noise reduction rate of the different approaches can be measured. The second region was chosen at an edge because the performance near the edges differs for the various approaches. Sometimes a lower noise reduction rate is achieved near higher contrast edges. Therefore, it is interesting to compare the noise reduction rates close to edges for different contrasts. Furthermore, the

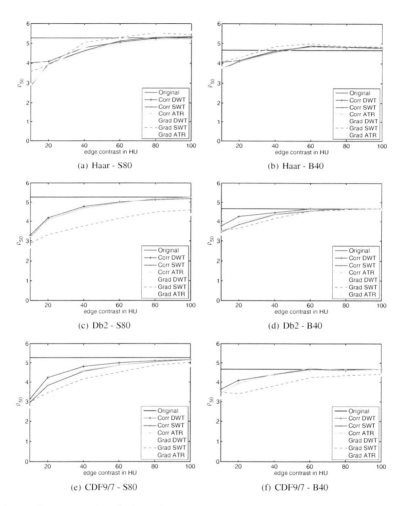

Figure 4.9: The ρ_{50} values in dependence on contrast at the edge for different methods and wavelets.

Table 4.1: Percentage noise reduction in a homogeneous image region.

S80	Grad			Corr		
	ATR	DWT	SWT	ATR	DWT	SWT
Haar	26.9	22.9	26.0	42.1	39.2	40.7
Db2	27.4	22.9	26.3	46.2	44.9	45.7
CDF9/7	27.6	23.2	26.5	48.2	47.9	48.1

B40	ATR	DWT	SWT	ATR	DWT	SWT
Haar	26.6	22.0	25.4	38.9	36.3	38.3
Db2	26.1	22.5	25.9	43.5	42.2	43.2
CDF9/7	27.0	22.7	26.2	45.5	44.9	45.4

noise reduction rates were evaluated for the two different reconstruction kernels (S80 and B40).

In the homogeneous image region, no noticeable changes are observed when the contrast of the objects is changed. Therefore, the measurements in cases of 100, 60 and 20 HU are averaged. Tab. 4.1 presents the noise reduction rates (percentage values) measured in the homogeneous image region. The first clear observation is that the noise suppression for the *Corr* method is much higher than that for the *Grad* method. The computation of correlation coefficients between pixel regions taken from the approximation images leads to smoother similarity measurements. This is also noticeable regarding the weighting matrices in Fig. 4.4 in comparison to Fig. 4.3.

An interesting observation is that, for the *Grad* method, the noise reduction rates do not vary for the different wavelets. In contrast to that, when using the *Corr* approach, slightly increased noise suppression can be achieved for longer reaching wavelets. By increasing the length of the wavelet filters, larger pixel regions are used for the similarity computations. This avoids the case where noisy homogeneous pixel regions are accidentally detected as correlated. In contrast, the fact that the approximated gradient vectors in noisy homogeneous pixel regions can sometimes point to the same direction cannot be reduced by using longer reaching wavelets. The comparison of the three wavelet transformation methods shows that DWT again has the lowest noise suppression capability, while SWT and ATR perform comparably. This shows that nonreducing wavelet transformations are better for noise suppression due to their inherent redundancy. All these observations can be made for both convolution kernels. The difference is, that in the images with lower noise level, due to the reconstruction with a smoothing kernel like the B40, the noise reduction rate is approximately 3 percent points in the case of the *Corr* method and less than 1 percent point in the case of the *Grad* method below the noise reduction rate in the more noisy images reconstructed with the S80.

Table 4.2 lists the noise reduction rates achieved in the edge region, again using the two different convolution kernels. Here, the results are compared for three different contrasts at the edge. Most of the observations for the homogeneous image region are also valid for the edge region. The *Corr* approach clearly outperforms the *Grad* method. The DWT shows the lowest noise suppression, whereas ART and SWT are comparable. In the case of the *Grad* method, it can be observed that there is nearly no differences between the different wavelets. Generally, with decreasing contrast at the edge, more noise in the local neighborhood of the edge can be removed. The reason for this is that the lower the contrast, the lower the influence of the edge to the correlation analysis. However, one difference between the two similarity computation methods becomes clear: For the *Grad* approach

Table 4.2: Percentage noise reduction rates in an edge region.

S80		Grad			Corr		
		ATR	DWT	SWT	ATR	DWT	SWT
100HU	Haar	25.4	21.2	24.1	38.4	35.3	37.0
	Db2	25.2	21.6	24.1	40.0	39.0	39.6
	CDF9/7	25.9	21.5	24.5	36.0	35.6	36.0
60HU	Haar	26.5	22.1	25.2	40.1	37.9	38.9
	Db2	26.6	21.6	24.8	42.1	41.1	41.8
	CDF9/7	27.0	21.7	25.4	39.0	38.0	38.9
20HU	Haar	26.6	21.7	25.1	40.7	38.1	39.4
	Db2	26.6	22.1	25.4	43.8	42.3	43.3
	CDF9/7	27.1	22.4	25.4	43.2	42.5	43.1

B40		ATR	DWT	SWT	ATR	DWT	SWT
100HU	Haar	22.9	19.8	22.4	33.0	31.1	32.6
	Db2	21.8	19.3	22.0	34.8	34.1	34.7
	CDF9/7	22.3	19.2	22.2	29.4	28.8	29.7
60HU	Haar	25.3	21.2	24.0	35.8	33.6	35.0
	Db2	24.4	19.6	23.1	37.7	36.5	37.4
	CDF9/7	25.3	19.9	23.7	32.7	31.7	32.6
20HU	Haar	25.1	20.3	24.0	36.0	34.1	35.4
	Db2	24.8	20.3	24.2	39.0	37.1	38.8
	CDF9/7	25.7	21.0	24.4	36.9	35.7	36.9

the increment in noise suppression with decreasing contrast at the edge is quite similar for all wavelets. This does not hold for the *Corr* approach. With increasing spatial extension of the wavelet filters, the difference between the noise reduction rate at 100 HU increases in comparison to 20 HU increases. This means that for higher contrast, more noise close to edges remains in the image if longer reaching filters are utilized. The reason for this is that the size of the pixel regions used for the correlation computations are adapted to the filter lengths of the wavelets. This is needed in order to ensure that all coefficients, which include information of an edge, are included in the similarity computations, as already mentioned during the discussion of Fig. 4.3. The effect is that edges with contrast highly above the noise level dominate the correlation computation, as long as they occur within the pixel region. As a result, nearly no noise is removed within a band around the edge. The width of the stripe obviously depends on the spatial extension of the wavelet filters.

Noise-Resolution-Tradeoff

Within the last two sections a very detailed, contrast dependent evaluation of noise and resolution was presented. For easier comparison of the different denoising approaches, noise-resolution-tradeoff curves are plotted in Fig. 4.10(a). The phantom described in Section 4.4.1 with an edge-contrast of 100 HU, reconstructed with the S80 kernel, was used for the experiment. The ρ_{50} values are plotted against the standard deviation of noise, measured within a homogeneous image region. The *Corr* and *Grad* method in combination with DWT, SWT and ATR are compared, all using the Db2 wavelet and 3 decomposition levels. The power p within the weighting function (Eq. (4.21)) was used for varying the amount of noise suppression. The 10 points within each curve correspond to the powers $p \in \{5.0, 4.5, 4.0, 3.5, 3.0, 2.5, 2.0, 1.5, 1.0, 0.5\}$ from left to right. In summary the following observations can be made:

- SWT and DWT show better edge-preservation than ATR at the same noise reduction rate in combination with the *Grad* method.

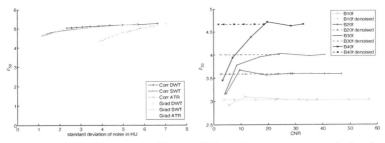

(a) Comparison of denoising methods with varying weighting functions.

(b) Comparison between reconstruction kernels.

Figure 4.10: Left: Noise-Resolution-Tradeoff: Comparison of high-contrast resolution and standard deviation of noise in homogeneous image region for different denoising methods using Db2 wavelet. The power p within the weighting function (4.21) is used for varying the amount of noise suppression. Right: Noise-Resolution-Tradeoff: ρ_{50} polotted against CNR for different reconstruction kernels. Denoising configuration: 3 level SWT with CDF9/7 wavelet and *Corr* method.

- The *Corr* method clearly outperforms the *Grad* method in all cases.

- There is nearly no difference between the different wavelet transformations if the *Corr* approach is used.

In a second test, the influence of the reconstruction kernel to the noise-resolution-tradeoff was evaluated. Different reconstruction kernels can be selected in CT, always leading to a noise-resolution-tradeoff. Smoothing reconstruction kernels imply lower noise power, but also lower image resolution. As already seen during the discussion of noise and resolution in the last two sections the reconstruction kernel also influences the results of the denoising method. Therefore, the noise-resolution-tradeoff is compared for different reconstruction kernels (see Fig. 4.7) with and without the application of the proposed denoising method. We used again the phantom images described in Section 4.4.1 with varying contrasts c, reconstructed with B10, B20, B30 and B40 kernel. The contrast-to-noise ratio (CNR $= c/\sigma$) and resolution (ρ_{50}) of the original and denoised images were then compared. A 3 level SWT with CDF9/7 wavelet and the *Corr* method was used for the comparison shown in Fig. 4.10(b). The dashed lines correspond to the original and the solid lines to the denoised images. Each line consists of six points corresponding to the contrasts (10, 20, 40, 60, 80 and 100 HU) divided by the respective standard deviation of noise σ measured in a homogeneous image region. Ideally the denoising procedure would only increase the CNR without lowering resolution. This would mean that the solid lines are just shifted to the right in comparison tho the corresponding dashed lines. The observed behavior, however, is more complex and corroborates the results presented in the previous sections:

- The sharper the kernel (high resolution, low CNR), the higher the improvement in CNR that can be achieved by applying the proposed method.

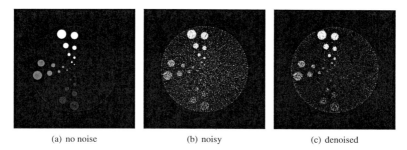

(a) no noise   (b) noisy   (c) denoised

Figure 4.11: Low-contrast-phantom (LCP) used for human observer study: (a) ideal noise-free, (b) one noisy example and (c) corresponding denoised image using 3 levels of SWT, CDF9/7 wavelet and the *Corr* method. Display options: $c = 5, w = 12$.

- The smoother the kernel (low resolution, high CNR), the better the edge-detection and thus the preservation of resolution in the denoised image.

The new insight gained from this analysis is that better results can be achieved with respect to image resolution and CNR using a sharper reconstruction kernel in combination with the proposed method than using a smoother reconstruction kernel. For example, higher resolution and higher CNR is obtained for the same input data if the sharper B30 kernel is used in combination with the proposed filter than using the smoother B10 kernel without denoising.

4.4.2 Low-Contrast-Detectability

In addition to the quantitative evaluation of noise and resolution a human observer study was performed. This allows to test, how the low-contrast-detectability is influenced by the application of the proposed method.

Data and Experiment

For the experiments reconstructions from a simulated cylindrical water phantom ($r = 14.5$ cm), with four blocks of embedded cylindrical objects with different contrasts (10, 5, 3, 1 HU) and different sizes ($15, 12, 9, 7, 5, 4, 3, 2$ mm diameter) were used. A reconstructed slice from this phantom is shown in Fig. 4.11(a). 10 noisy realizations of this phantom were simulated and reconstructed, all at the same dose level ($30\,\mathrm{mAs}$), leading to an average pixel noise in the homogeneous water region of $\sigma = 4.3\,\mathrm{HU}$. One noisy example slice is shown in Fig. 4.11(b). In addition to this, 20 noisy phantoms were simulated, where some (95 in sum) of the embedded objects were missing. The same scanning and reconstruction parameters were used for all 30 datasets. For all 30 images the corresponding denoised images (with approx. 44% noise reduction, leading to $\sigma = 2.4\,\mathrm{HU}$ in average) were computed. 3 decomposition levels of SWT in combination with CDF9/7 wavelet together with the *Corr* method were used. As an example, in Fig. 4.11(c) the denoised image of Fig. 4.11(b) can be seen.

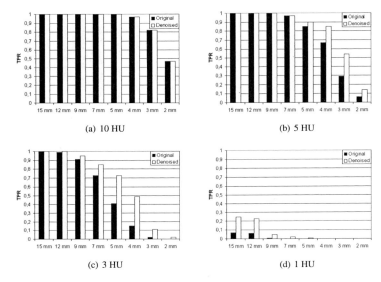

(a) 10 HU

(b) 5 HU

(c) 3 HU

(d) 1 HU

Figure 4.12: Comparison of true-positive rates for different objects of noisy (original) and denoised LCP.

For easier accomplishment and evaluation of the experiment a proprietary evaluation tool for low-contrast-detectability was developed. This tool shows the images from a list in randomized order to the human observer. The observer then has to select which objects he can detect by mouse click. All 47 observers (most of them PhD students in the field of medical image processing) evaluated 40 images, 10 original noisy images where all objects were present, the 10 corresponding denoised, 10 noisy images where some objects were missing, and again the 10 corresponding denoised.

Results and Discussion

In a first step the average true-positive rate (TPR) achieved for the different objects was evaluated. The performance of detecting objects of different size and contrast was compared between the noisy and denoised images. The average TPR was computed for all 32 objects from all noisy images and all observers and compared to the average from all denoised images and all observers. In Fig. 4.12 the TPR is plotted for all objects of different contrasts and sizes. The closer the TPR is to 1 the better the object was correctly judged to be visible in average. The clear result is that all objects were judged to be as well or even better visible in the denoised images in comparison to the noisy originals. The corresponding false-positive rates (FPR) are all below 0.03 and in average below 0.005 for both noisy and denoised images. In Fig. 4.12(a) the TPR for the 10 HU objects can be seen, where no clear difference between the noisy and denoised objects is visible. In case of the 5 HU and 3 HU objects (see Fig. 4.12(b) and 4.12(c)) a clear difference can be seen. If objects with a TPR above 0.5 are said to be detectable, two more objects (5 HU, 3 mm and 3 HU, 5 mm)

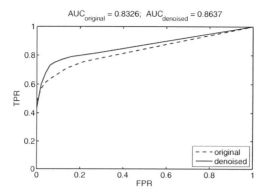

Figure 4.13: ROC curves resulting from human observer study. Comparison between noisy (original) and denoised results.

are detectable in the denoised images than in the noisy ones. The TPR of the $3\,\mathrm{HU}, 4\,\mathrm{mm}$ object is also very close to 0.5. The $1\,\mathrm{HU}$ objects are nearly never detected in the noisy images, but in the denoised at least the 15 and 12 mm objects are detected correctly in more than 20% of the cases.

In a second step, receiver operating characteristic (ROC) curves for the noisy and denoised cases based on a thresholding approach were computed, as described in detail in [Fawc 06]. Firstly, the average detection rate (number of positive votes that object is visible / number of overall votes for this object) was computed for each single image and object from all observers. Then, a sliding threshold was applied for the noisy and denoised cases separately. All objects with a detection rate above a certain threshold were set to be detected and then the corresponding FPR and TPR was calculated, leading to the curves shown in Fig. 4.13. In addition to the curves the area under the curve (AUC) was computed for the noisy and denoised case. The AUC improved from 0.8326 in case of the noisy to 0.8637 in case of the denoised samples.

4.4.3   Comparison with Adaptive Filtering of Projections

Data and Description

Fig. 4.14 shows a comparison of the proposed method to a projection based adaptive filtering, which is used in clinical practice [Brud 01]. The 2-D-projections are filtered with a linear filter of fixed spatial extension. Then, a weighted sum of the filtered and original noisy projections is computed based on the attenuation at a respective position. The higher the attenuation, the higher the noise power and, therefore, the stronger the smoothing being performed. This method, like most other noise reduction methods based on filtering the projections, has the goal to reach nearly constant noise variance over all projections in order to reduce directed noise.

For the comparison reconstructions from two simulated elliptical phantoms were used, one homogeneous water phantom ($r = 10\,\mathrm{cm}$) and one eccentric water phantom ($a =$

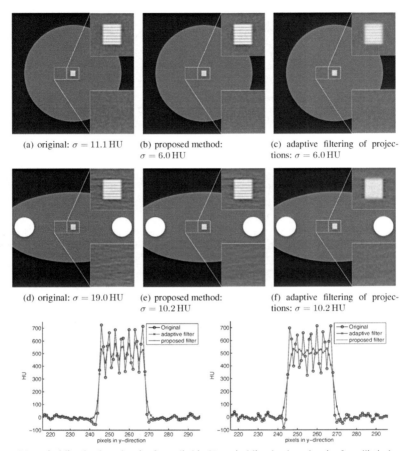

(a) original: $\sigma = 11.1\,\text{HU}$ (b) proposed method: $\sigma = 6.0\,\text{HU}$ (c) adaptive filtering of projections: $\sigma = 6.0\,\text{HU}$

(d) original: $\sigma = 19.0\,\text{HU}$ (e) proposed method: $\sigma = 10.2\,\text{HU}$ (f) adaptive filtering of projections: $\sigma = 10.2\,\text{HU}$

(g) vertical lineplot through noise-free cylindrical phantom, proposed(b) and adaptively filtered projections(c)   (h) vertical lineplot through noise-free elliptical phantom, proposed(e) and adaptively filtered projections(f)

Figure 4.14: Comparison of proposed method to adaptive filtering of projections. The reconstruction without noise suppression are displayed in (a) and (d). The proposed wavelet based noise reduction method was applied in (b) and (e) and the adaptive filtering of the projections is shown in (c) and (f). Image resolution of the filtered images is compared at the same noise reduction rates. In (g) and (h) the corresponding vertical lineplots through the center of the two phantoms are compared between the noise-free, adaptive-filtered and wavelet denoised images. Display options: $c = 200$ and $w = 1000$.

15 cm and $b = 7.5$ cm). In the center of both phantoms a line-pattern with $6\,\mathrm{lp/cm}$ is embedded at a contrast of $1000\,\mathrm{HU}$. In the eccentric phantom two additional cylindrical objects ($r = 2$ cm) are embedded. All reconstructions to a pixel grid of 512×512 with FOV of 25 cm were performed using the B40 kernel. In Fig. 4.14(a) and Fig. 4.14(d) the original noisy phantoms reconstructed from the complete set of projections are shown. The standard deviation of noise was measured in homogeneous regions in north, south, west and east direction around the center resulting in an average noise of $\sigma = 11.1\,\mathrm{HU}$ in the homogeneous, and $\sigma = 19.0\,\mathrm{HU}$ in the eccentric water phantom. Both denoising methods were applied to achieve the same average noise reduction rate, leading to $\sigma = 6.0\,\mathrm{HU}$ in the homogeneous and $\sigma = 10.2\,\mathrm{HU}$ in the eccentric case, and resolution is compared. For the proposed method, 3 levels of SWT together with the CDF9/7 wavelet and the *Corr* method was used.

Results and Discussion

Fig. 4.14(f) shows that directed noise pointing out the direction of highest attenuation is reduced. A remarkable noise suppression can be achieved by adaptively filtering the projections. However, it can also be seen by visual inspection that structures orthogonal to the direction of highest attenuation lose spatial resolution. In comparison to this the wavelet based filtering method preserves structures much better. No blurring effects are visible. This can be seen well in the detailed vertical lineplots through the line-pattern, shown in Fig. 4.14(g). Although the same average noise reduction rate is obtained, the noise streaks are not completely removed using the wavelet approach. This is the strength of the adaptive filtering method. In contrast to this, the adaptive filtering method does not perform well if rotationally symmetric objects are present. The goal of the adaptive filtering of the projections is to achieve nearly constant noise variance over all projections. If the noise variance is already very similar in all projections, the adaptive filtering does nothing at all, or loses resolution in all directions. This can be seen well in Fig. 4.14(c). Here, the wavelet based method, as shown in Fig. 4.14(b), can again achieve a high noise reduction rate without loss of resolution. The detailed vertical lineplots are again shown in Fig. 4.14(h). Nevertheless, it should be emphasized that the noise suppression based on projection is a pre-processing step, i. e. prior to reconstruction, while the proposed method is a post-processing step, thus making the combination of the two methods possible.

4.4.4 Clinically Acquired Data

Data and Experiment

In order to test the noise reduction method with respect to its practical usability, the application of the algorithm on clinically acquired data is indispensable. Noise reduction methods are particularly critical in their application to low contrast images. Thus, images predominantly including soft tissue are well suited for performance assessment. Theoretically, as already discussed, the higher the contrast of edges, the higher the probability that the edge can be detected and preserved. If the application of the method with specific parameter settings leads to good results in slices with soft tissue, the use for higher contrast regions will not be critical. Therefore, a thoraco-abdomen scan (see examples in Fig. 4.16), acquired with a Siemens Sensation CT-scanner, was used for the clinical evaluation. The reconstruction of slices at a FOV of 38 cm with a thickness of 3 mm was performed with a B40 kernel, which is one of the standard kernels for this body region.

For the clinical experiment, 12 noise-suppressed images were computed from the same input images with different configurations. Three different wavelet transformation methods (ATR, DWT and SWT) in combination with two different wavelets (Haar and CDF9/7) were utilized. Furthermore, these configurations together with the *Corr* and *Grad* methods for similarity computation were compared. The resulting noise-reduced images and the average of the input images, which corresponds to the reconstruction from all projections, were compared by a radiologist. All images correspond to the same dose level. For simple comparison, a proprietary evaluation tool was developed. A randomized list of comparisons between image pairs can be performed with this tool. Within each comparison, an image pair is shown to the radiologist. The initial position of the two images is also randomized. However, the positions of the two images can be easily switched by the radiologist, in order to facilitate the detection of even very small differences between the images. The radiologist decides if there is one preferred image (clear winner) or both images are judged of equal quality with respect to the following evaluation criteria.

Three different quality criteria were evaluated separately in three consecutive tests:

- detectability of anatomical structures,

- noise in homogeneous image regions,

- noise in edge regions.

In each test, all possible image pairs were compared to each other. Altogether, 3×78 comparisons were performed. The outcome of these tests is shown in Fig. 4.15. The dark bars show the number of clear winners, normalized to the number of performed comparisons for one image. The corresponding light bars are the results of a score system. Three points are gained by a winning image and one point if two images are judged to be of equal quality. This value is again normalized, this time to the number of maximally reachable points, if the image won all comparisons.

Results and Discussion

In the first test (Fig. 4.15(a)), the detectability of anatomical structures was examined. Only in one case the anatomical structures were judged to be better detected in the original image than in the noise suppressed image. In all other direct comparisons of noise reduced images to the average of input images (here denoted as original), the processed images were chosen to be favorable. This shows that the anatomical structures are well preserved by the noise suppression method. The separation of information and noise is further improved because of the better signal-to-noise ratio. The comparison between the different configurations shows that the *Corr* method gives better edge detection results than the *Grad* approach. There is no clearly preferred wavelet basis or wavelet transformation.

In the second test (Fig. 4.15(b)), the treatment of noise in homogeneous image regions was analyzed. Here again, the *Corr* method gives much better visual results in all cases. There is nearly no difference between the Haar and the CDF9/7 wavelet.

In the final test (Fig. 4.15(c)), the noise in regions around edges was compared. This test reflects the results of the quantitative evaluation with phantom data. It shows that nearly

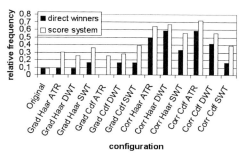

(a) Detectability of anatomical structures

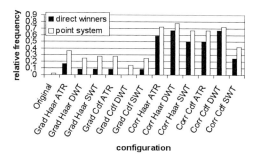

(b) Noise in homogeneous image region

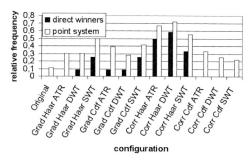

(c) Noise in edge region

Figure 4.15: Results of the clinical evaluation - (a) Detectability of anatomical structures; (b) noise in homogeneous regions and (c) noise in edge regions were compared for different configurations.

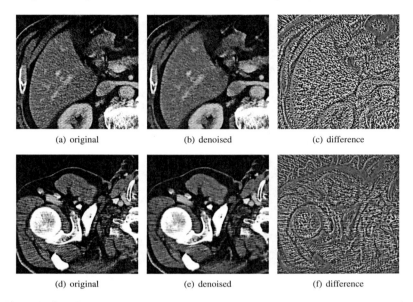

(a) original   (b) denoised   (c) difference

(d) original   (e) denoised   (f) difference

Figure 4.16: Noise suppression in clinical images from the abdomen (a)-(c) and thorax (d)-(f). Configuration: SWT, Haar wavelet, $l_{max} = 3$, $p = 1$, *Corr* method. Display options: $c = 50$, $w = 400$ for CT-images and $c = 0, w = 50$ for difference images.

no noise is removed in regions of edges if long reaching wavelets are used in combination with the *Corr* method. The results of the Haar wavelet are still judged better for the *Corr* method in comparison to the *Grad* approach.

The *Corr* method is clearly preferred considering the results of all three tests together. However, longer reaching wavelets lead to lower noise reduction around higher contrast edges. Therefore, a tradeoff between smoothness and spatial locality of the wavelet must be resolved.

4.4.5   Example Images

Two examples of noise suppression on clinically acquired data are shown in Fig. 4.16. Zoomed-in images from the abdomen (4.16(a)-4.16(c)) and thorax (4.16(d)-4.16(f)) are displayed. For denoising, 3 levels of a Haar wavelet decomposition (SWT) in combination with the *Corr* method were used. The original images, which correspond to the reconstruction from the complete set of projections, are compared to the noise suppressed images. Additionally, the differences between the original and denoised images are shown. Noticeably, noise in homogeneous image regions is removed, while structures are well preserved.

In Fig. 4.17 two examples of a thorax-abdomen phantom acquired at a Siemens Definition dual-source CT (DSCT) scanner are shown. We used the same scan protocol

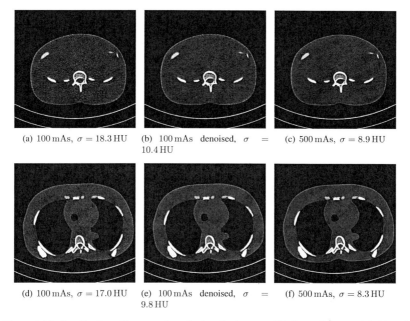

(a) 100 mAs, $\sigma = 18.3$ HU

(b) 100 mAs denoised, $\sigma = 10.4$ HU

(c) 500 mAs, $\sigma = 8.9$ HU

(d) 100 mAs, $\sigma = 17.0$ HU

(e) 100 mAs denoised, $\sigma = 9.8$ HU

(f) 500 mAs, $\sigma = 8.3$ HU

Figure 4.17: Application of proposed method to dual-source CT data: abdomen (a)-(c) and thorax (d)-(f). Configuration: SWT, Db2 wavelet, $l_{max} = 3$, $p = 1$, *Corr* method. Display options: $c = 50$, $w = 300$.

(100 mAs, 120 kV, slice-thickness= 1.2 mm) and reconstruction parameters (FOV= 35 cm, kernel = B30) for both source-detector systems. The image reconstructed from projections acquired at the first detector is denoted as A and the image from the second detector is denoted as B. The FOV (26 cm) of the second detector is smaller than that of the first detector. Therefore, the projections of the B-system are extended at the outer borders with data from the A-system, as explained in detail in [Brud 06]. With this technique two images can be reconstructed at the full FOV. Inside the 26 cm-FOV independent acquisitions from the two detectors are available. Consequently, noise within these regions can be assumed to be uncorrelated between the two images. Outside the FOV of 26 cm only parts of the projections derive from independent measurements due to the padding. Therefore, noise in this outer region is no longer perfectly uncorrelated. Evaluating the correlation during the *Corr* method or comparing the angle between the approximated gradient vectors in the *Grad* method still works in this outer region. However, only a lower noise reduction can be achieved because of the increasing correlation between A and B with increasing distance from the 26 cm radius. In Fig. 4.17(a) and Fig. 4.17(d) the average images of A and B are shown for two examples. The A and B images are then used as input to the proposed noise reduction method (3 levels SWT with Db2 wavelet and *Corr* method). The corresponding denoised results are shown in Fig. 4.17(b) and Fig. 4.17(e). For better comparison high-dose scans (500 mAs) are shown in Fig. 4.17(c) and Fig. 4.17(f). Within the overlapping FOV, where data from both detectors has been acquired, a noise reduction rate of approximately 43% was achieved. Due to the sinogram extension of the B-system with data from A, noise outside the FOV of 26 cm is no longer perfectly uncorrelated. Therefore, only a lower noise reduction of approximately 25% can be achieved in regions outside the overlapping FOV.

4.5 Conclusions

In this chapter a robust and efficacious wavelet domain denoising technique for the suppression of pixel noise in CT-images was introduced. The separate reconstruction from disjoint subsets of projections allows the generation of images which only differ with respect to image noise but include the same information. A correlation analysis based on the detail coefficients of the á-trous wavelet decomposition of the input images, as recently proposed by Tischenko, allows the separation of structures and noise, without assuming or estimating the underlying noise distribution. An extension of Tischenko's approach for the applicability with DWT and SWT was described. The quantitative and qualitative evaluation showed that comparable edge preservation, with only slightly lower noise reduction, can also be achieved with DWT at lower computational costs. Best results with respect to noise and resolution evaluation can be obtained using the non-redundant SWT. More importantly, a second similarity measurement was introduced which makes use of correlation coefficients. Weighting of wavelet coefficients according to the correlation coefficient based similarity measurement shows improved results with respect to edge preservation and noise suppression for all wavelet transformations. In addition to the contrast dependent noise and resolution evaluation, human observer tests were performed for evaluating the low contrast detectability. The performed human-observer study showed that the detectability of small low-contrast objects could be improved by applying the proposed method. In comparison to a commonly applied projection based algorithm, the proposed method achieved higher resolution at the same noise suppression. The evaluation on clinically-acquired CT data proves the practical usability of the methods.

Chapter 5

Noise Estimation in the Wavelet Domain for Anisotropic Noise Reduction

The approaches proposed in the last chapter automatically adapt themselves to the local noise in the image because of the local correlation analysis between two separately reconstructed images. Especially in homogeneous image regions high noise reduction rates of about 45% can be achieved. It is a problem that noise very close to edges sometimes visibly remains. Further, if images with strongly directed noise due to high absorption along certain directions are processed, a compromise between noise reduction and edge-preservation must be found. No anisotropic noise reduction can be performed, where noise along edges is removed without smoothing across the edges. The reason for this can be found in weighting all three blocks of detail coefficients based on the same weighting image. In this section another wavelet based noise reduction approach is presented, which has partially been published in [Bors 08d]. The method is based on wavelet thresholding, as it has first been proposed by Donoho and Johnstone [Dono 94]. The idea of wavelet thresholding is to erase insignificant detail coefficients below a defined threshold and preserve those with larger values. The noise suppressed image is obtained by an inverse wavelet transformation from the modified coefficients. The difficulty is to find a proper threshold, especially for noise of spatially varying power and directed noise, which is commonly present in CT-images. Choosing a very high threshold may lead to visible loss of image structures, but the effect of noise suppression may be insufficient, if the chosen threshold was too low. Therefore, a reliable estimation of noise for threshold determination is one of the main issues.

The main contributions presented in this chapter can be summarized as follows: The method is again based on two separately reconstructed CT datasets. This time the two datasets are used for local noise estimation. The coherences of the noise variance between different linear combinations of separately reconstructed images is described. Based on the difference between the two input datasets the variance of noise in the input images and in the mean image can be estimated. Due to the linearity of the wavelet transformation, the same theory can be applied: The noise variance of the wavelet coefficients can be estimated from the difference of the wavelet coefficients of the input images. Noise adaptive thresholds are computed for detecting insufficient detail coefficients and suppressing them by hard thresholding.

5.1 Methodology Overview

An overview of the proposed noise reduction method is shown in Fig. 5.1. First, two images A and B are generated, which only differ with respect to image noise. The generation of two input images, which only differ with respect to noise, has already been described in Section 4.2. Each of the images is then decomposed by a two dimensional wavelet transformation. The redundancy included in the stationary wavelet transformation (SWT) is advantageous for reducing noise [Coif 95]. Also the investigation in Chapter 4 showed best noise reduction in CT in combination with SWT. Therefore, the discussion in this section is restricted to SWT. The computation of the differences between the detail coefficients of the two input images A and B shows just the noise in the respective frequency band and orientation. These noise images can be used for the estimation of the position and orientation dependent noise variances in A and B. From these estimates, a thresholding mask is computed and applied to the wavelet coefficients of the image reconstructed from the complete set of projections. In case of a linear CT-reconstruction method the thresholds are directly applied to the averaged detail coefficients of the input images. The computation of the inverse wavelet transformation using the modified coefficients results in a noise-suppressed image. This again corresponds to the reconstruction from the complete set of projections but with improved signal-to-noise ratio.

5.2 Noise Estimation for Adaptive Thresholding

In this section the theoretical background for the noise estimation is described. First, the variance of noise in a linear combination of the input images is investigated. The coherence between noise in the difference image and the mean image builds the basis for noise estimation in the wavelet domain. The second part introduces how the noise estimation can be used for computing local, frequency and orientation dependent thresholds and how to apply those to the detail coefficients of the wavelet representation of the input images.

5.2.1 Noise Estimation from Difference Image

Two images A and B are reconstructed from disjoint subsets of projections. In the following, we assume that the sampling theorem is fulfilled for both subsets of projections. Noise between the projections can be assumed to be uncorrelated, if crosstalk at the detector is negligibly small. Consequently, A and B only differ with respect to image noise, but include the same ideal noise-free signal:

$$A = S + N_A, \quad B = S + N_B, \tag{5.1}$$

where $S = \mathcal{E}(A) = \mathcal{E}(B)$ represents the ideal noise-free image (the statistical expectation $\mathcal{E}$) and $N_A \neq N_B$ zero-mean noise ($\mathcal{E}(N_A) = \mathcal{E}(N_B) = 0$) included in image A and B, respectively. Noise in both images is non-stationary, and consequently the noise variance depends on the local position $\mathbf{x} = (x, y)^T$. The variances at a given pixel position are approximately the same in both images:

$$\sigma_A^2(\mathbf{x}) \approx \sigma_B^2(\mathbf{x}), \tag{5.2}$$

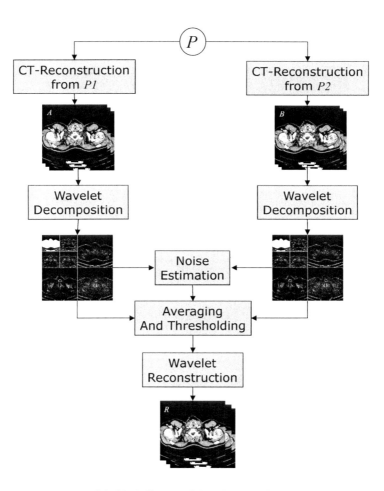

Figure 5.1: Block diagram of the noise reduction method.

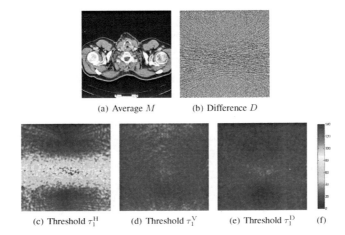

(a) Average M (b) Difference D

(c) Threshold τ_1^H (d) Threshold τ_1^V (e) Threshold τ_1^D (f)

Figure 5.2: Example of orientation and position dependent threshold at the first decomposition level for thoracic image with strongly directed noise. The average of input images is shown in (a) and their difference in (b). The threshold images in horizontal (c), vertical (d) and diagonal (e) directions were computed with $k = 1.0$ and $s = 4$. The color-mapping is shown in (f).

because on average the same number of contributing quanta can be assumed. Noise between the projections P1 and P2 is uncorrelated and accordingly noise between the separately reconstructed images is uncorrelated, too, leading to the following covariance:

$$\mathrm{Cov}(N_A, N_B) = 0. \tag{5.3}$$

The linear combination L of A and B is defined as:

$$L = g_1 A + g_2 B, \tag{5.4}$$

with weights $g_1, g_2 \in \mathbb{R}$. For the variance of a linear combination of random variables the following holds [Bron 00]:

$$\sigma_L^2 = g_1^2 \sigma_A^2 + g_2^2 \sigma_B^2 + 2g_1 g_2 \mathrm{Cov}(A, B). \tag{5.5}$$

It can be shown that

$$
\begin{aligned}
\mathrm{Cov}(A, B) &= \mathcal{E}((A - \mathcal{E}(A))(B - \mathcal{E}(B))) \\
&= \mathcal{E}((A - S)(B - S)) \\
&= \mathcal{E}(N_A \cdot N_B) \\
&= \mathrm{Cov}(N_A, N_B) - \mathcal{E}(N_A)\mathcal{E}(N_B) \\
&= 0.
\end{aligned}
\tag{5.6}
$$

Using Eq. (5.2) and Eq. (5.6), Eq. (5.5) results in:

$$\sigma_L = \sqrt{g_1^2 + g_2^2}\, \sigma_A. \tag{5.7}$$

First of all, Eq. (5.7) shows why the noise level in A and B is increased by a factor of $\sqrt{2}$ in comparison to the reconstruction from the complete set of projections or the average of the two input images $M = \frac{1}{2}(A + B)$. Furthermore, it can be used for estimating noise in A and B and consequently in M from the difference of the input images. By the computation of the difference image

$$D = A - B = N_A - N_B,\qquad(5.8)$$

a noise-image free of structures is obtained. Based on Eq. (5.7), the standard deviations σ_A and σ_B of noise can be approximated from the standard deviation in the difference image σ_D by:

$$\sigma_A = \sigma_B = \frac{\sigma_D}{\sqrt{2}}.\qquad(5.9)$$

Thus, the standard deviation of noise in the average image M results in:

$$\sigma_M = \frac{\sigma_A}{\sqrt{2}} = \frac{\sigma_D}{2}.\qquad(5.10)$$

5.2.2 Adaptive Thresholding

In order to compute a level and orientation dependent threshold for denoising in the wavelet domain, noise in the different frequency bands and orientations should be estimated separately. Due to the known linearity of the wavelet transformation, the differences between the detail coefficients can also be directly used for noise estimation. At each decomposition level l the difference images

$$
\begin{aligned}
D_l^{\mathrm{H}}(\mathbf{x}) &= W_{A,l}^{\mathrm{H}}(\mathbf{x}) - W_{B,l}^{\mathrm{H}}(\mathbf{x}), & (5.11)\\
D_l^{\mathrm{V}}(\mathbf{x}) &= W_{A,l}^{\mathrm{V}}(\mathbf{x}) - W_{B,l}^{\mathrm{V}}(\mathbf{x}), & (5.12)\\
D_l^{\mathrm{D}}(\mathbf{x}) &= W_{A,l}^{\mathrm{D}}(\mathbf{x}) - W_{B,l}^{\mathrm{D}}(\mathbf{x}) & (5.13)
\end{aligned}
$$

between the detail coefficients are computed, where the subscripts A and B correspond to the respective image and H, V and D again denote the horizontal, vertical and diagonal directions. These difference images are then used for the estimation of noise in the respective frequency band and orientation. In CT-images, the noise power is spatially varying. Therefore, noise estimation should be position dependent. The standard deviation of noise is evaluated in quadratic local neighborhoods of given size in the difference images. Averaging over local neighborhoods always implies an ergodicity assumption, which is not fulfilled in case of CT, but is necessary for getting more reliable noise estimates from the difference images. We estimate the standard deviation σ_l^d at decomposition level l in the direction $d \in \{\mathrm{H, V, D}\}$ according to:

$$\sigma_l^d(\mathbf{x}) = \sqrt{\frac{1}{|\Omega_{\mathbf{x}}|} \sum_{\tilde{\mathbf{x}} \in \Omega_{\mathbf{x}}} (D_l^d(\mathbf{x}))^2}.\qquad(5.14)$$

The local square pixel region $\Omega_{\mathbf{x}}$ centered around the current position $\mathbf{x} = (x, y)^T$ is defined as:

$$\Omega_{\mathbf{x}} = \left\{ \tilde{\mathbf{x}} \big| \, |x - \tilde{x}| \le s \wedge |y - \tilde{y}| \le s \right\},\qquad(5.15)$$

where the constant s defines the size of the quadratic pixel region. The number of pixels used for the local noise estimation is denoted as $|\Omega_\mathbf{x}|$. Analogously, the noise estimates for the vertical and diagonal directions are computed. From the three standard deviation images σ_l^H, σ_l^V and σ_l^D, for all decomposition levels, orientation and position dependent thresholds are determined according to:

$$\tau_l^\mathrm{H}(\mathbf{x}) = k\,\frac{\sigma_l^\mathrm{H}(\mathbf{x})}{2} \tag{5.16}$$

$$\tau_l^\mathrm{V}(\mathbf{x}) = k\,\frac{\sigma_l^\mathrm{V}(\mathbf{x})}{2}$$

$$\tau_l^\mathrm{D}(\mathbf{x}) = k\,\frac{\sigma_l^\mathrm{D}(\mathbf{x})}{2}$$

The constant k controls the amount of noise suppression. With increasing k the thresholds are increased. Consequently, more coefficients are set to zero and more noise is removed. In Fig. 5.2(c)-5.2(e) the thresholds computed with $s = 4$ for the first decomposition level in the horizontal, vertical and diagonal directions are shown for a thorax-slice (see average of input images in Fig. 5.2(a) with strongly directed noise (see difference of input images in Fig. 5.2(b)).

The computed thresholds from Eq. (5.16) are then applied to the averaged wavelet coefficients of the input images:

$$W_{M,l}^\mathrm{H}(\mathbf{x}) = \frac{1}{2}(W_{A,l}^\mathrm{H}(\mathbf{x}) + W_{B,l}^\mathrm{H}(\mathbf{x})), \tag{5.17}$$

$$W_{M,l}^\mathrm{V}(\mathbf{x}) = \frac{1}{2}(W_{A,l}^\mathrm{V}(\mathbf{x}) + W_{B,l}^\mathrm{V}(\mathbf{x})),$$

$$W_{M,l}^\mathrm{D}(\mathbf{x}) = \frac{1}{2}(W_{A,l}^\mathrm{D}(\mathbf{x}) + W_{B,l}^\mathrm{D}(\mathbf{x})).$$

We perform a *hard* thresholding, meaning that all averaged coefficients with an absolute value below the threshold are set to zero and values above are kept unchanged. The high frequency detail coefficients of the result image are computed as:

$$W_{R,l}^d(\mathbf{x}) = \begin{cases} W_{M,l}^d(\mathbf{x}), & \text{if } \left|W_{M,l}^d(\mathbf{x})\right| \geq \tau_l^d(\mathbf{x}), \\ 0, & \text{else} \end{cases} \tag{5.18}$$

for all directions $d \in \{\mathrm{H, V, D}\}$ and decomposition levels $l = 1 \ldots l_{\max}$. The approximation coefficients $A_{l_{\max}}$ and $B_{l_{\max}}$ of A and B at the maximum decomposition level $l_{\max}$ are simply averaged:

$$R_{l_{\max}}(\mathbf{x}) = \frac{1}{2}(A_{l_{\max}}(\mathbf{x}) + B_{l_{\max}}(\mathbf{x})). \tag{5.19}$$

The final noise suppressed image is computed by an inverse wavelet transformation from the averaged and weighted wavelet coefficients of the input images.

5.3 Experimental Evaluation

The evaluation section consists of two parts. In the first part, the noise estimation method based on the difference between two separately reconstructed CT images is evaluated. The second part concentrates on the performance evaluation of the proposed wavelet based noise reduction method.

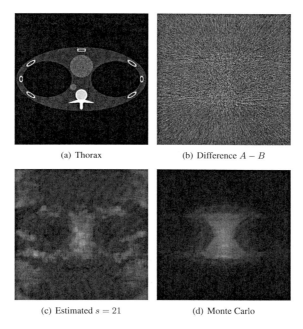

(a) Thorax   (b) Difference $A - B$

(c) Estimated $s = 21$ (d) Monte Carlo

Figure 5.3: Thorax phantom used for evaluation of noise estimation accuracy, reconstructed with Sim50 (30 cm FOV, display: w=50,c=400), together with analytical noise estimates and estimates from 10000 noisy realizations (Noise Display: w=25,c=50).

5.3.1 Accuracy of Noise Estimates

The estimation of the local standard deviation of noise in reconstructed CT images might also be of interest for other post-processing applications besides the here proposed adaptive filtering method. Therefore, in this section the noise estimation based on the difference between two separately reconstructed CT images is evaluated. For this purpose, two standard phantoms were simulated and reconstructed:

- The FORBILD thorax phantom, in the following denoted as thorax phantom, is shown in Fig. 5.3(a), reconstructed at a FOV of 41 cm, of slice positioned at $z = 0$ cm.

- The FORBILD head phantom with ears is shown in Fig. 5.4(a), reconstructed at a FOV of 25 cm, of slice positioned at $z = 0$ cm.

For both phantoms, noise-free fan-beam projections were simulated using 1160 projection, 672 detector channels and quarter detector offset. The following physical parameters were selected for the simulation: focus width 0.7 mm, anode angle $-82°$, delta beta $360/4640$ mm, sub delta beta 25, 80 kV. For the experiments three reconstruction kernels, a smooth (Sim10), a medium sharp (Sim30) and sharp (Sim50) one, were used. For the

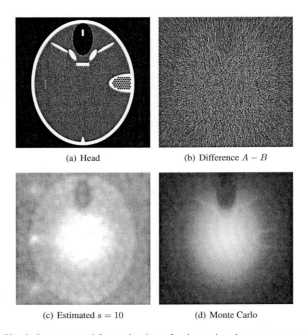

(a) Head   (b) Difference $A - B$

(c) Estimated $s = 10$ (d) Monte Carlo

Figure 5.4: Head phantom used for evaluation of noise estimation accuracy, reconstructed with Sim50 (25 cm FOV, display: w=50,c=900), together with analytical noise estimates and estimates from 10000 noisy realizations (Noise display: w=50,c=150).

noise estimation based on the proposed method, two noise realizations were generated. Poisson-distributed noise was added to the projections, in both cases using half of the overall dose. The reconstructions from the two noise realizations were then used for the computation of the difference image that served as a basis for the noise estimation within local neighborhoods of different sizes ($s = 4, 6, 8, 10$). The standard deviation image computed according to the proposed method is denoted as $\sigma_a(\mathbf{x})$. In order to generate a gold standard of the standard deviation image, Monte-Carlo simulation with $N_{MC} = 10000$ CT images was performed. For each image Poisson-distributed noise was added to the projections, this time using the overall dose. Pixel-wise noise computation from the N_{MC} reconstructed images gives $\sigma_b(\mathbf{x})$ the gold standard to compare with.

Examples for the computed standard deviation images and the Monte-Carlo results are presented in Fig. 5.3 and Fig. 5.4. For a better comparison of the noise estimates, horizontal and vertical lineplots through the standard deviation images of the gold standard and the computed estimates with different sizes of pixel regions s are presented in Fig. 5.5. From the lineplots it can already be seen that for large FOVs, where the sampling theorem is no longer fulfilled, the sampling-artifacts influence the noise estimation results. Aliasing artifacts or sampling-artifacts appear in both separately reconstructed images and are usually not uncorrelated, leading to high values in the difference images. If artifacts are dominant compared to the noise level in the image, the standard deviation of noise might be strongly over-estimated. This is clearly noticeable in the lineplots presented in Fig. 5.5 at the outer borders of the large FOV used in case of the thorax phantom. In the following, the quantitative evaluation is restricted to the inner FOV (here: 20 cm), where sampling-artifacts are not noticeable. This part of the image domain is in the following denoted as Ω_i and $N_i = |\Omega_i|$ denotes the number of image pixels inside of Ω_i. The pixelwise relative error is defined as:

$$r_\Delta(\mathbf{x}) = \frac{\sigma_a(\mathbf{x}) - \sigma_b(\mathbf{x})}{\sigma_b(\mathbf{x})}. \tag{5.20}$$

The noise propagation method is precise if the relative pixelwise errors are small inside Ω_i. Therefore, the average relative error

$$\bar{r}_\Delta = \frac{1}{N_i} \sum_{\mathbf{x} \in \Omega_i} r_\Delta(\mathbf{x}), \tag{5.21}$$

and its variance

$$\sigma_{r_\Delta}^2 = \frac{1}{N_i - 1} \sum_{\mathbf{x} \in \Omega_i} (r_\Delta(\mathbf{x}) - \bar{r}_\Delta)^2, \tag{5.22}$$

over the different image pixels is computed. The average error, normalized on a per-pixel basis is defined as:

$$s_\Delta = \sqrt{\frac{1}{N_i} \sum_{\mathbf{x} \in \Omega_i} (r_\Delta(\mathbf{x}))^2} = \sqrt{(\bar{r}_\Delta)^2 + \frac{N_i - 1}{N_i} \sigma_{r_\Delta}^2}. \tag{5.23}$$

Tab. 5.1 summarizes the results achieved for the two phantoms. The average pixel noise values σ_b in HU are listed for the two phantoms and three reconstruction kernels. The quantitative evaluation shows that pixelwise relative L2-norm errors between 11.6% and 20.7% are achieved with the proposed method for the two phantoms under investigation. A noise estimation based on just two measurements, thus only allows a rough estimation

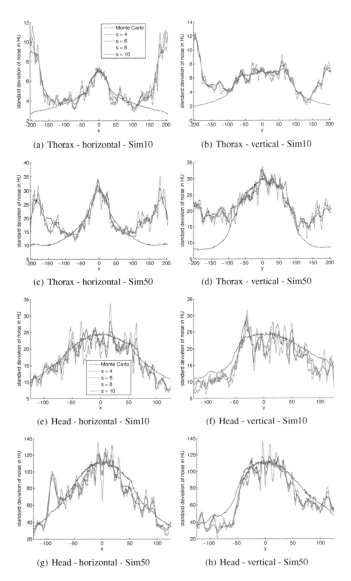

Figure 5.5: Horizontal and vertical cuts through standard deviation images for thorax phantom and head phantom - comparison of Monte-Carlo results to noise estimation results within different sizes of neighborhoods for two different reconstruction kernels.

Table 5.1: Evaluation of the error of the noise estimation method within a 20 cm FOV. Errors are quoted in percent (%).

Thorax - Sim10	$s = 4$	$s = 6$	$s = 8$	$s = 10$
$\bar{\sigma}_b$	19.4	19.4	19.4	19.4
r_Δ	-5.1±17.4	-4.5±13.9	-4.2±12.0	-4.0±10.9
s_Δ	18.1	14.6	12.7	11.6
Thorax - Sim30	$s = 4$	$s = 6$	$s = 8$	$s = 10$
$\bar{\sigma}_b$	31.6	31.6	31.6	31.6
r_Δ	-7.9±16.0	-7.3±13.0	-7.0±11.5	-6.8±10.7
s_Δ	17.8	14.9	13.5	12.7
Thorax - Sim50	$s = 4$	$s = 6$	$s = 8$	$s = 10$
$\bar{\sigma}_b$	64.8	64.8	64.8	64.8
r_Δ	-9.9±12.6	-9.6±11.2	-9.4±11.2	-9.4±10.5
s_Δ	18.6	16.0	14.8	14.1
Head - Sim10	$s = 4$	$s = 6$	$s = 8$	$s = 10$
$\bar{\sigma}_b$	18.8	18.8	18.8	18.8
r_Δ	-9.3±18.4	-8.5±13.9	-8.2±11.5	-8.0±9.9
s_Δ	20.7	16.3	14.1	12.8
Head - Sim30	$s = 4$	$s = 6$	$s = 8$	$s = 10$
$\bar{\sigma}_b$	31.0	31.0	31.0	31.0
r_Δ	-11.2±15.2	-10.7±12.1	-10.5±10.5	-10.4±9.7
s_Δ	18.9	16.1	14.9	14.2
Head - Sim50	$s = 4$	$s = 6$	$s = 8$	$s = 10$
$\bar{\sigma}_b$	74.7	74.7	74.7	74.7
r_Δ	-11.1±14.0	-10.8±11.9	-10.7±10.8	-10.6±10.0
s_Δ	17.9	16.6	15.2	14.6

of the pixelwise standard deviation of noise. In order to make the noise estimates more reliable, the standard deviation is computed in local neighborhoods of certain sizes s. With increasing size of the pixel regions used for evaluating the local standard deviation in the difference image, the results get smoother, but also less local, as expected. For the relative error, it can be seen that only a slight improvement is noticeable with increasing size of the pixel regions s. It is of course important to notice that with this averaging over a certain neighborhood, ergodicity is assumed. Ergodicity implies that averaging over a certain spatial region has the same effect as averaging over a certain number of realizations. Even if noise in the reconstructed CT image varies slowly over the different pixel regions, noise in the reconstructed CT images is not uncorrelated, which makes the noise estimation based on the evaluation within local neighborhoods less reliable. The effect of averaging over the neigborhood is also influenced by the size of the noise grains in comparison to the size of the pixel region. The more uncorrelated values can be averaged, the more reliable gets the noise estimate. Generally, one would expect that with smoother reconstruction kernels the number of correlated values within a fixed sized pixel region increase and thus the noise estimate gets worse. The comparison between the different reconstruction kernels shows that this effect is only noticable for smaller pixel regions. For $s = 4$ the noise estimates improve the sharper the reconstruction kernel is. On the other hand with increasing sharpness of the reconstruction kernel noise changes faster between different pixels. Therefore, the non-local noise estimation due to averaging over a pixel region has a more severe influence, when sharp reconstruction kernels are used. If the L2-norm errors are compared between the differen reconstruction kernels, using $s = 10$, the noise estimates get less reliable on a per-pixel basis if sharper kernels are used. Further, with decreasing FOV the number of correlated pixels within a fixed size region increase, also making the noise estimates less reliable. This effect is noticeable comparing the results of the thorax phantom and head phantom. The head phantom was reconstructed at a smaller FOV, resulting in a smaller

pixel size. Consequently, more pixels withnin a certain fixed sized pixel region are correlated in case of the head phantom compared to the thorax phantom. The noise estimates
achieved for the head phantom at the same size of pixel region and the same reconstruction
kernel are thus less reliable.

The noise estimation based on the difference between two separately reconstructed
noise realizations is not very reliable and is sometimes affected by reconstruction artifacts.
However, the big advantage of the proposed method is that it is fast, easy to implement
and that it can also be extended to be used for estimating noise in the wavelet domain
of the images. The evaluation in the next section will show that it is much better to use
the proposed rough noise estimation for the computation of local, frequency and orientation dependent thresholds than using standard wavelet filtering approaches, where global
frequency dependent thresholds are estimated.

5.3.2   Noise and Resolution

The second part of the evaluation section considers the proposed wavelet based noise reduction method. In evaluating the performance of the noise reduction method, mainly
two aspects are of interest: the amount of noise reduction and, even more importantly, the
preservation of anatomical structures. Therefore, the influence of the noise suppression
method to the standard deviation of noise and image resolution was investigated.

For the experiments reconstructions from a simulated elliptical water phantom ($dx =
20\,\text{cm}$, $dy = 10\,\text{cm}$), with an embedded, quartered cylinder ($r = 6\,\text{cm}$) with a contrast of
$100\,\text{HU}$ were used. The projections P1 and P2 were simulated independently, corresponding to two consecutive scans or the acquisition with a dual-source-scanner. The advantage
of simulations is that in addition to noisy projections (with Poisson distributed noise according to quantum statistics), ideal, noise-free data can also be produced. All slices are of
size 512×512 and were reconstructed using the indirect filtered backprojection reconstruction described in Section 2.2.2 within a field of view of $20\,\text{cm}$ using a sharp Shepp-Logan
filtering kernel. This results in an average pixel noise of approximately $22.4\,\text{HU}$ in the
homogeneous image region in the reconstruction from the complete set of projections. The
standard deviation of noise in the separately reconstructed images is about $\sqrt{2}$ times higher.

All images were denoised with the proposed thresholding method up to the fourth decomposition level of a Haar-SWT. The size of the pixel region defined in Eq. (5.15) was
set fixed to $s = 4$. Different values of $k \in \{1, 1.5, 2, 2.5, 3\}$ were used for regulating the
amount of noise suppression. The proposed method was compared to a standard wavelet
thresholding approach implemented in the Matlab Wavelet Toolbox[Wave 06]. For denoising in Matlab, we used a *Balance Sparsity-Norm* hard thresholding method with a
non-white-noise model and again four levels of a Haar-SWT. Further, the proposed thresholding approach was compared to the edge-preserving noise reduction method presented
in the last chapter Chapter 4, where the weights at each decomposition level were gained
from a correlation analysis between the approximation images of the previous decomposition level. Again four decomposition levels of a Haar-SWT were used the correlations were
computed within neighborhoods of 5×5 pixels around the corresponding position. The
amount of noise suppression was controlled by the power within the weighting function
Eq. (4.21), denoted by parameter $p \in \{1, 1.5, 2, 2.5, 3\}$. In the following we use the ab-

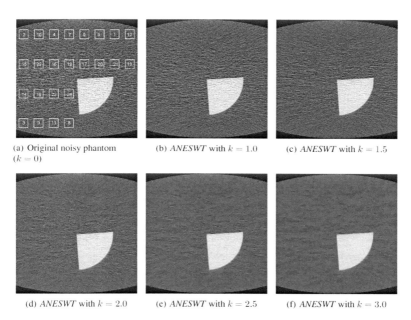

(a) Original noisy phantom ($k = 0$) (b) *ANESWT* with $k = 1.0$ (c) *ANESWT* with $k = 1.5$

(d) *ANESWT* with $k = 2.0$ (e) *ANESWT* with $k = 2.5$ (f) *ANESWT* with $k = 3.0$

Figure 5.6: Phantom used for noise and resolution evaluation. (a) Original noisy phantom, where regions used for noise evaluation are marked. (b)-(f) Denoised images achieved with proposed method (*ANESWT*) with different values of parameter k controlling the amount of noise suppression. Center and window settings used for displaying CT-images: c=50, w=200.

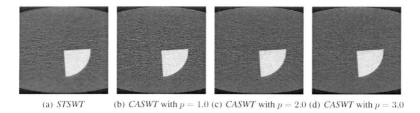

(a) *STSWT* (b) *CASWT* with $p = 1.0$ (c) *CASWT* with $p = 2.0$ (d) *CASWT* with $p = 3.0$

Figure 5.7: Denoising results achieved with standard wavelet thresholding (*STSWT*) (a) and correlation analysis based wavelet denoising (CASWT) (b)-(d) for different values of parameter p controlling the amount of noise suppression. Center and window settings used for displaying CT-images: c=50, w=200.

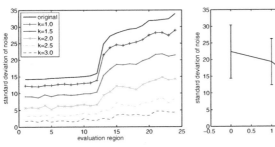

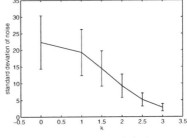

(a) Standard deviation of noise

(b) Mean noise and standard deviation between regions

Figure 5.8: Noise evaluation for *ANESWT* in different pixel regions marked in Fig. 5.6(a). (a) Comparison of standard deviation of noise in different pixel regions for different values of k. (b) Mean standard deviation of noise of all pixel regions together with standard deviation between different pixel regions for different values of k.

breviation *STSWT* for the standard thresholding, *CASWT* for the correlation analysis based denoising method, and *ANESWT* for the proposed adaptive noise estimation based method.

In Fig. 5.6 the used noisy phantom together with the denoised images achieved with *ANESWT* for different values of k is shown. Due to the eccentricity of the used phantom, directed noise is clearly visible, pointing out in the direction of highest attenuation. This can be seen in the original noisy image in Fig. 5.6(a). For better comparison, the denoising results achieved with *STSWT* and *CASWT* for different values of p are presented in Fig. 5.7. In order to compare the noise homogeneity before and after denoising, the standard deviations of noise were evaluated in 24 homogeneous image regions of 40×40 pixels as marked in Fig. 5.6(a). The standard deviations of noise in the different pixel regions are plotted in Fig. 5.8(a) for the original and the denoised images using *ANESWT*. The pixel regions are numbered incrementally according to their standard deviation of noise in the original image. It can be seen that with increasing k stronger noise suppression is achieved, as expected. Furthermore, it can be seen that, with increasing k, noise between the different evaluation regions becomes more homogeneous. This is even clearer in Fig. 5.8(b), where the average standard deviations of noise from all evaluation regions are plotted for the different values of k ($k = 0$ denotes the original image), together with the standard deviations between the 24 evaluation regions. As Fig. 5.8(b) shows, with increasing k not only the average noise in the image is reduced, but also the standard deviation between the pixel regions is decreased.

Fig. 5.9(c) shows the noise evaluation for *STSWT*. In all pixel regions the standard deviation of noise was decreased. However, it can be seen that the algorithm does not adapt to the noise level in the image. Regions with a higher noise level are not stronger denoised. Fig. 5.9(a) shows the noise evaluation for *CASWT*. The average standard deviation of noise together with the standard deviation between the different pixel regions is shown in Fig. 5.9(b). With increasing parameter p a stronger noise suppression is achieved. The direct comparison of the standard deviations of noise in the different pixel regions between *ANESWT* and *CASWT* shows that a comparable noise suppression in pixel regions 1-12

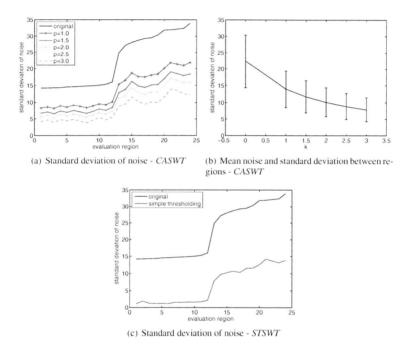

(a) Standard deviation of noise - *CASWT*   (b) Mean noise and standard deviation between regions - *CASWT*

(c) Standard deviation of noise - *STSWT*

Figure 5.9: Noise evaluation for *CASWT* (a) and (b) and *STSWT* (c). The same pixel regions were used, as marked in Fig. 5.6(a). (a) Comparison of standard deviation of noise in different pixel regions for different values of p. (b) Mean standard deviation of noise of all pixel regions together with standard deviation between different pixel regions for different values of p. (c) Standard deviation of noise in different pixel regions.

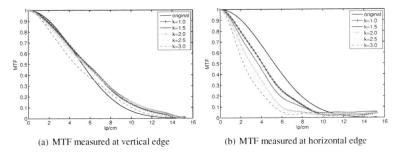

(a) MTF measured at vertical edge   (b) MTF measured at horizontal edge

Figure 5.10: Evaluation of image resolution for *ANESWT*. MTFs of vertical (c) and horizontal (d) edge are compared for different values of k.

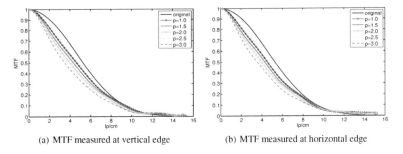

(a) MTF measured at vertical edge   (b) MTF measured at horizontal edge

Figure 5.11: Evaluation of image resolution for *CASWT*. MTFs of vertical (c) and horizontal (d) edge are compared for different values of p.

is e.g. achieved for $k = 2.0$ and $p = 2.0$. In contrast to that, the average noise suppression in pixel regions 13-24 achieved with $k = 2.0$ approximately corresponds to that achieved with $p = 2.5$. *ANESWT* reduces more noise in regions with strong directed noise. Consequently, a lower standard deviation between the different pixel regions is achieved.

For evaluating image resolution the local modulation transfer function (MTF) was again evaluated at an edge. In order to achieve reliable measurements, the MTF was again evaluated in the modified noise-free images. The computed thresholds at each decomposition level are applied to the wavelet coefficients of the ideal noise-free image followed by an inverse wavelet transformation. This has the effect of making the influence of the weighting to the real signal directly visible. The local MTF can then be computed at the edge in the processed noise-free image. In Fig. 5.10 MTFs computed from the horizontal and vertical edge can be seen. In Fig. 5.10(a) it can be seen that the vertical edge was very well preserved. Image resolution at the vertical edge could even be improved. The increment in resolution, when using the Haar wavelet, has already been discussed in the last chapter in Section 4.4. In contrast to the high resolution at the vertical edge, a slight blurring is noticeable at the horizontal edge, as can be seen Fig. 5.10(b). In Fig. 5.11 the resolution evaluations performed for *CASWT* are shown. Here, it can be observed that there is nearly no difference with respect to edge-preservation for the horizontal and vertical edge.

5.3.3 Example Images

In Fig. 5.12(d) and Fig. 5.12(f), zoomed-in noise-suppressed results from the proposed method applied to a thoracic image (see Fig. 5.2(a)) are shown for two different settings of k. The two input datasets A and B were generated by separate reconstructions from even and odd numbered projections. The difference images (Fig. 5.12(e), 5.12(g)) between the denoised and average of input images (Fig. 5.12(a)) are also displayed. The images are compared to the denoising result achieved with the *SWT De-noising 2-D* tool from the Matlab wavelet toolbox [Wave 06] (see Fig. 5.12(b) and 5.12(c)). All computations were performed using a Haar wavelet decomposition up to the fourth decomposition level. For denoising in Matlab, we used a *Balance Sparsity-Norm* hard thresholding method with a non-white-noise model.

The difference image in Fig. 5.12(c) shows that standard wavelet thresolding methods reduce noise in the images, but also blur edges. The reason for this is that no reliable noise estimation is possible if just one CT-image is available. In contrast, the proposed method adapts itself to the spatially varying noise power in the different frequency bands and orientations and, therefore, performs much better especially in images with directed noise.

5.4 Conclusions

In this chapter an anisotropic wavelet domain denoising technique for the suppression of pixel noise in CT-images was proposed. The separate reconstructions from disjoint subsets of projections allows the generation of images which only differ with respect to image noise but include the same ideal noise-free signal. A new approach for estimating noise in the different frequency bands and orientations of the wavelet transformation, based on the difference between the wavelet coefficients of the two separate reconstructions, was proposed. With this technique, position and orientation adaptive thresholds can be computed at each decomposition level for noise reduction.

The experiments show that standard denoising techniques like *STSWT* lead to unconvincing results if they are applied to CT images. The reason for this can be found in the difficult noise properties in CT. The noise distribution after reconstruction is not known, noise is non-stationary and directed noise may be present. This makes the distinction between real structures and noise more complicated. The presented examples, where *STSWT* was applied to CT slices with directed noise, clearly showed that in regions of higher noise level noise still remains in the image, while other regions already get blurred.

The *CASWT*, another wavelet based method for noise suppression on CT data, presented in Chapter 4, showed that an adaptation to the noise level is performed. The method adapts itself to the noise level of the input data by computing the local correlations between the wavelet representations of two separately reconstructed CT images. At each decomposition level, one weighting image is computed. This is applied equally to the different directions. Therefore, this method does not allow anisotropic denoising. In images

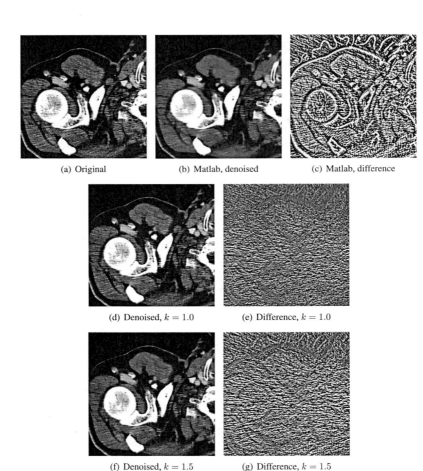

(a) Original   (b) Matlab, denoised   (c) Matlab, difference

(d) Denoised, $k = 1.0$ (e) Difference, $k = 1.0$

(f) Denoised, $k = 1.5$ (g) Difference, $k = 1.5$

Figure 5.12: Denoising result of the proposed method (d),(f) in comparison to standard wavelet thresholding method from the Matlab wavelet toolbox (b) in pixel region taken from a thorax-slice with strongly directed noise (a). The corresponding difference images to the original (a) are displayed in (c),(e) and (g). Center and window settings used for displaying CT-images: c=50, w=400. Center and window settings used for displaying difference images: center=0, window=30.

with strong directed noise, a higher noise suppression always influences the resolution in horizontal and vertical direction in the same way.

The proposed thresholding method adapts itself to the local and orientation dependent noise power in CT. In contrast to *CASWT*, the proposed *ANESWT* performs an anisotropic noise reduction. Noise is estimated separately within the different frequency bands and orientations of the wavelet decomposition. The thresholds used for denoising are chosen in adaptation to the local noise estimates. Consequently, locally varying and also directed noise can be removed efficiently. The evaluation of noise in different pixel regions showed that stronger denoising is performed where stronger directed noise is present. This has the effect that not only the overall noise power is reduced, but also the standard deviation between the different evaluation regions is decreased. Thus, the homogeneity of noise within the image is improved. The anisotropic behavior of the proposed method can also be observed in the evaluation of resolution. With *ANESWT*, stronger smoothing is performed orthogonal to the direction of the directed noise. This is the reason why with increasing k stronger blurring is visible at the horizontal than at the vertical edge. In comparison to *CASWT* the blurring at the horizontal edge is slightly increased. However, the vertical edge is nearly perfectly preserved, also at high noise reduction rates. The anisotropic behavior is beneficial, especially in cases where directed noise due to high attenuation along certain directions is present.

The experiments performed on clinical data showed that directed noise could be removed without noticeable loss of resolution with the new denoising approach. Especially, the difference images between the original and denoised images show that nearly no structure was removed. Further, it can be seen that noise along edges could also be removed. The comparison to *STSWT* applied to clinical data again showed that no reliable estimation of locally-varying and directed noise can be achieved if just one input image is available. In the example shown, noise was strongly over-estimated resulting in noticeable blurring at the edges.

The proposed method is computationally efficient. The cost for reconstructing the two datasets A and B separately corresponds a reconstruction from the complete set of projections. Two reconstructions each with only half the number of projections are needed, if only the even or odd numbered projections are used respectively. Otherwise, if the object is scanned twice or a dual-source-scanner is used two complete reconstructions are needed. The denoising process can be computed efficiently. There are two wavelet decompositions and one inverse wavelet transformation to be computed. The complexity of the SWT is linear with the number of pixels. All computations needed for weighting the coefficients are performed within local neighborhoods. Thus, the method is well suited for parallel computation.

Chapter 6

Multiple CT-Reconstructions for 3-D Anisotropic Wavelet Denoising

Two different approaches for noise reduction in the wavelet domain based on two input datasets have been proposed in the last two chapters. It has been shown that the two input datasets and respectively their wavelet representations can be utilized for local correlation analysis and noise estimation. This chapter presents an approach that combines the both previous methods and has partially been published in [Bors 07b].

The main contributions in this chapter can be summarized as follows: A correlation analysis between the approximation coefficients of the two input datasets, combined with an orientation and position dependent noise estimation is used for differentiating between structure and noise. Furthermore, the extension of the method to 3-D is investigated, which additionally leads to a more reliable correlation analysis and noise estimation.

6.1 Methodology Overview

An overview of the methodology can be found in Fig. 6.1. First two volumes A and B are reconstructed from disjoint subsets of projections. The generation of two datasets, which only differ with respect to noise, but include the same ideal noise-free signal, has already been described in Section 4.2. Also the noise properties in CT and in separately reconstructed datasets has been discussed in detail in Section 5.2. These properties are considered during the denoising process proposed here, which can be applied either to the 2-D slices or the 3-D volumes. Both datasets are decomposed by a 2-D or 3-D discrete dyadic wavelet transformation. After this linear transformation, for example of the input dataset $A = A_0$, four two-dimensional or eight three-dimensional blocks of coefficients are available at each decomposition level l: the lowpass filtered approximation A_l and the highpass filtered details W_l^d, where d describes the direction in space. For the 2-D case, e.g., d can be the horizontal, vertical or diagonal direction. The detail coefficients include high frequency structures together with noise in the respective frequency bands and orientations. In the following the wavelet representations of the two input datasets are used for differentiating between detail coefficients that belong to structure and noise, and to compute weighting coefficients accordingly. These weights consist of two parts: a correlation coefficient based weight and a significance-weight, which are both described more in detail in the following section. The computed weights are then applied to the

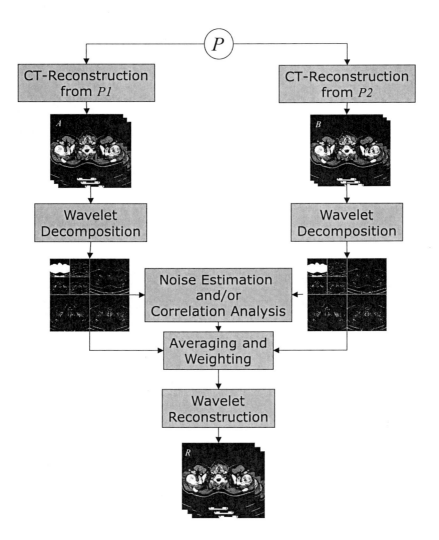

Figure 6.1: Block diagram of the noise reduction method.

wavelet coefficients of the reconstruction from the complete set of projections. In case of a linear reconstruction method, this corresponds to the averaged wavelet coefficients of the input datasets. It is, thus, ensured that the entire acquired data is used for the final result R, which is computed by an inverse wavelet transformation from the modified coefficients.

6.2   3-D Wavelet Transformation

The computation of higher-dimensional wavelet transformations is a straight forward extension of the one-dimensional case. As explained in Section 3.4.1 the one dimensional transformation is successively applied in all dimensions, what is called separable wavelet transformation. The separable extension can be applied to the DWT as well as to the SWT. Working with volumes, however, makes the whole processing more complicated due to the increased memory consumption. If CT volumes with nearly isotropic resolution in all three spatial dimensions are generated, several hundreds of two-dimensional slices are usually computed. In most cases, the two complete separately reconstructed volumes do not fit completely into the main memory. Therefore, the complete stack of images is split into smaller blocks that are large enough for the computation of the wavelet transformation up to the maximum decomposition level but fit into the main memory. Another consideration that is also closely related to the memory problem is the restriction of the 3-D case to DWT. Although, it has been shown before that the redundant SWT has some advantages with respect to denoising purposes compared to the DWT, the storage complexity is very high for the 3-D-SWT. All eight blocks of 3-D detail coefficients that are computed at each decomposition level have the same size as the original volume to be decomposed. If, e. g., l_{max} levels of a SWT are computed in 3-D, the number of wavelet coefficients are factor $8l_{max} + 1$ larger than the number of samples in the original volume. This is not practicable for the large volumes considered in case of CT. In the following of this chapter the wavelet decomposition is, therefore, restricted to the DWT.

6.3   Anisotropic Denoising Using Correlation Analysis

The detail coefficients of the two input datasets contain structure and noise in the respective frequency bands and orientations. The goal is to detect coefficients that represent structure and keep them. Other noisy coefficients should be suppressed. The distinction between structures and noise is here, based on a local correlation analysis and noise estimation.

6.3.1   Correlation Analysis

At each decomposition level, a local correlation analysis between the approximation coefficients of A and B is performed. This leads to one block of correlation coefficients having the same size as the detail coefficients at the respective decomposition level l.

A very close connection between the detail coefficients and the correlation analysis can be obtained if the approximation coefficients of the previous decomposition level $l - 1$ are used for correlation analysis at level l. The detail coefficients at level l are computed from the approximation coefficients at level $l - 1$ and these values are also used for correlation analysis at the respective position. For the correlation based weight $G_l^{cor}(\mathbf{x})$, the empirical correlation coefficient $C_l(\mathbf{x})$ is computed according to Eq. (4.7). Approximation coefficients A_{l-1} and B_{l-1} within a local neighborhood $\Omega_\mathbf{x}$ around the corresponding position in the approximation are used. The correlation value is then mapped to the interval $[0, 1]$. Altogether, the correlation base weight at the position $\mathbf{x}$ is computed according to Eq. (4.19):

$$G_l^{\text{corr}}(\mathbf{x}) = \frac{1}{2}\left(C_l(\mathbf{x}) + 1\right)^p \in [0, 1]. \tag{6.1}$$

6.3.2   Noise Estimation

Additionally, for each orientation a local noise estimation is computed in order to assess the significance of each detail coefficient versus the noise level.

The difference $D = A - B = N_A - N_B$ between the two input datasets shows just noise. Due to the linearity of the wavelet transformation the difference of the wavelet coefficients can be used for estimating the local and orientation dependent standard deviation of noise in the different frequency bands of the wavelet decomposition, as described in Chapter 5. The differences between the detail coefficients are computed for all decomposition levels $l = 1, \ldots, l_{\max}$ and all orientations d:

$$W_{D,l}^{\text{d}}(\mathbf{x}) = W_{A,l}^{\text{d}}(\mathbf{x}) - W_{B,l}^{\text{d}}(\mathbf{x}). \tag{6.2}$$

From these differences the corresponding standard deviations $\sigma_l^{\text{d}}(\mathbf{x})$ are locally computed for all positions $\mathbf{x}$ according to:

$$\sigma_l^{\text{d}}(\mathbf{x}) = \sqrt{\frac{1}{n}\sum_{\mathbf{x}\in\Omega_\mathbf{x}}(W_{D,l}^{\text{d}}(\mathbf{x}))^2}. \tag{6.3}$$

From this estimation, significance-weights are computed for each detail coefficient:

$$G_l^{\text{sig,d}}(\mathbf{x}) = \begin{cases} 1, & \left|W_{M,l}^{\text{d}}(\mathbf{x})\right| \geq k\sigma_l^{\text{d}}(\mathbf{x}), \\ e^{-\left(1-\left(\frac{W_{M,l}^{\text{d}}(\mathbf{x})}{k\sigma_l^{\text{d}}(\mathbf{x})}\right)^2\right)^r}, & \text{otherwise} \end{cases} \tag{6.4}$$

where $k \in \mathbb{R}, k \geq 0$ is a weighting factor. Averaged detail coefficients $W_{M,l}^{\text{d}}(\mathbf{x})$ with absolute value above the local, noise dependent threshold $k\sigma_l^{\text{d}}(\mathbf{x})$ are kept unchanged, values below are attenuated according to their difference to the threshold. The parameter k controls the amount of noise suppression in relation to the noise power. The higher the value of k, the more noise is removed. With increasing parameter $r \in \mathbb{R}$ the significance weight tends more and more to an adaptive hard thresholding. In our experiments we used $r = 10$.

6.3.3   Weighting of Detail Coefficients

Altogether, the averaged detail coefficients of A and B are weighted with the product of correlation based weight and significance-weight:

$$W_{R,l}^{\text{d}}(\mathbf{x}) = W_{M,l}^{\text{d}}(\mathbf{x}) \cdot G_l^{\text{sig,d}}(\mathbf{x}) \cdot G_l^{\text{corr}}(\mathbf{x}) \tag{6.5}$$

for all directions d and all decomposition levels $l = 1, \ldots, l_{\max}$. The approximation coefficients at the maximum decomposition level $l_{\max}$ are just averaged:

$$R_{l_{\max}}(\mathbf{x}) = \frac{1}{2}(A_{l_{\max}}(\mathbf{x}) + B_{l_{\max}}(\mathbf{x})). \tag{6.6}$$

The noise suppressed result R is obtained by an inverse discrete wavelet transformation of the averaged and weighted coefficients.

6.4 Experimental Evaluation

For the evaluation of the combined wavelet based filtering approach, experiments on simulated and measured data were performed. In the first part of the evaluation, noise and resolution were investigated based on simulated data. The amount of noise reduction and capability of preserving edges was compared for different configurations of the algorithm. Furthermore, a quantitative comparison between 2-D and 3-D denoising was performed. In the second part of the evaluation, example images are presented and a qualitative comparison of 2-D and 3-D results is performed.

6.4.1 Noise and Resolution

The proposed noise reduction method takes into account the local noise variance, the noise anisotropy and orientation. It is, therefore, important for the evaluation to use a phantom that on the one hand has enough variation in the local noise variance, but also shows clearly anisotropic noise characteristics. Reconstructions from a simulated elliptical water phantom (40 cm, 20 cm), with an embedded cylinder (radius 2.5 cm placed 10 cm off-center) were used for the noise and resolution analysis. With this phantom, on the one hand, the average standard deviation of noise within a certain region of interest can be evaluated. On the other hand, the circular object can be used for computing the average modulation transfer function on the edge of the circular inlay, as described in Section 2.5.2. Like for most adaptive nonlinear methods, the performance of the proposed algorithm with respect to the detection and preservation of real structures in the presence of noise, depends on the local contrast-to-noise level. Therefore, the contrast of the embedded object in comparison to water was varied (20, 60, 100 and 1000 HU), while the dose of radiation was kept constant, leading to different contrast-to-noise levels at the edge of the inlay. The dose of radiation, meaning the number of photons at the source, was chosen such that a standard deviation of noise in the image close to the cylinder of about 20 HU was obtained. Fan-beam projections with 672 channels and 1160 projections per full rotation were simulated. Noise-free projections were simulated first. For all contrast-to-noise levels 16 noisy realizations were generated by adding Poisson distributed noise to the projections. The A and B images were computed from the full number of projections each after adding Poisson distributed noise of half the overall dose to the projections. The generation of the input datasets, therefore, corresponds to acquiring the same object twice, or, using a dual-source CT scanner under ideal conditions. With ideal conditions we mean that both, the A- and B-system of the DSCT scanner cover the complete FOV. Furthermore, effects like photon scattering are neglected. All images were reconstructed at a FOV of 30 cm with the indirect fan-beam FBP method described in Section 2.2 using a medium sharp reconstruction kernel (Sim30).

The problem of evaluating the resolution in an image is that the contrast of the edge compared to the noise level must be high enough in order to achieve smooth MTF curves. The noise reduction method, however, behaves differently for varying contrast-to-noise levels, what makes a contrast dependent analysis necessary. In order to still achieve smooth MTF curves, the computed weights were again applied to the noise-free reconstructed image, as described in the previous two chapters. By weighting the wavelet coefficients of the noise-free reconstructed image, according to the weights computed from a certain pair of noisy A and B images, the influence of the processing to the ideal signal can be made visible. The results computed from weighting based on 16 different pairs of noisy input datasets A and B were additionally averaged before computing the MTF on the circular inlay. It should be reminded here that the computed MTF from a reconstructed CT image is not a modulation transfer function in the sense that it describes a linear shift-invariant system. It is more to be seen as a local average measurement for the resolution in the image. Especially, if the MTF is computed on the edge of the circular inlay, it is the average MTF of all the points on the circle surface and, additionally, an average over the certain different directions, because the profile of the edge is circularly averaged. In case of a linear system the MTF directly can be used for also determining the effect of the linear system on the standard deviation of noise. However, in case of an adaptive filtering and the computation of local MTFs it is necessary to evaluate the noise properties of the filter based on another figure of merit.

Of course, the figure of merit that describes, how well the method is reducing noise in the image should not be done completely without considering image resolution. A fair comparison of algorithms can only be achieved, if the noise level is compared for the same resolution, or the other way round. It is however, very difficult, especially for nonlinear adaptive methods, to tune the parameters such that exactly the same image resolution is achieved after filtering. Therefore, a new evaluation strategy is proposed here, that tries to do the noise evaluation under consideration of the local MTF measured from the image.

From the MTF measured on the edge of the circle a corresponding linear shift-invariant filter can be computed that leads to the same average smoothing in the image as the adaptive filter achieved in average on the edge of the circular inlay. Then the standard deviation of noise after adaptive filtering in comparison to standard deviation of noise after application of the linear filter that leads to the same average resolution at the inlay can be investigated. The frequency response of the one-dimensional linear filter $\hat{h}_{\mathrm{lfil}}(\rho)$ is computed from the quotient of the MTF ($\mathrm{MTF}_{\mathrm{afil}}(\rho)$) measured in the processed image and the original MTF ($\mathrm{MTF}_{\mathrm{orig}}(\rho)$) that is computed in a noise-free reconstruction of the phantom:

$$\hat{h}_{\mathrm{lfil}}(\rho) = \begin{cases} \frac{\mathrm{MTF}_{\mathrm{afil}}(\rho)}{\mathrm{MTF}_{\mathrm{orig}}(\rho)} & \text{if } \mathrm{MTF}_{\mathrm{afil}}(\rho) < \mathrm{MTF}_{\mathrm{orig}}(\rho) \text{ and } \mathrm{MTF}_{\mathrm{orig}}(\rho) \neq 0 \\ 1 & \text{otherwise} \end{cases}. \tag{6.7}$$

The MTF in the adaptively filtered image is here bounded by the original MTF. An increment of resolution at the edge is not accounted here. In order to achieve a linear shift-invariant and rotationally symmetrical filtering in two-dimensions, the reconstruction kernel is modified, by multiplying its frequency response $\hat{k}(\rho)$ with the frequency response of the linear filter:

$$\hat{k}_{\mathrm{mod}}(\rho) = \hat{k}(\rho)\hat{h}_{\mathrm{lfil}}(\rho). \tag{6.8}$$

The image corresponding to the linearly filtered version of a noisy image is obtained from another indirect fan-beam FBP reconstruction, but using the modified kernel $\hat{k}_{\mathrm{mod}}(\rho)$.

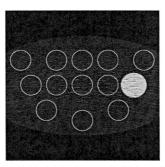

(a) Original noisy image with ROIs used for noise evaluation.

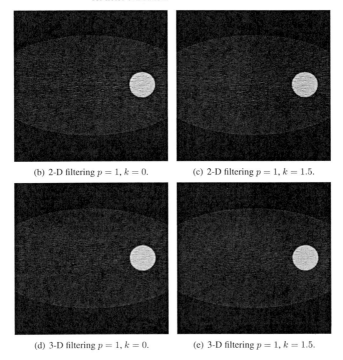

(b) 2-D filtering $p = 1$, $k = 0$.   (c) 2-D filtering $p = 1$, $k = 1.5$.

(d) 3-D filtering $p = 1$, $k = 0$.   (e) 3-D filtering $p = 1$, $k = 1.5$.

Figure 6.2: Elliptical water phantom with circular inlay (here with contrast of 100 HU) used for noise and resolution analysis. The regions used for noise evaluation are marked in the original noisy image (a). The results of filtering in 2-D without (b) and with consideration of significance weights (c) are compared to the filtering result achieved in 3-D without (d) and with significance weights (e). Display: c=50, w=200.

The standard deviation of noise is then evaluated in 12 homogeneous circular regions of the elliptical phantom, as displayed in Fig. 6.2(a). The standard deviation of noise is computed separately for all 12 regions for the original noisy image (σ_{orig}), the image filtered with the adaptive filter (σ_{afil}) and the image reconstructed with the linear filter that leads to the average same smoothing at the edge of the circular inlay (σ_{lfil}). The mean and the standard deviation of the noise standard deviations over the different image regions can thus be considered. For all image regions, the noise reduction rate achieved with the adaptive filter is defined as:

$$\mathrm{NRR} = 1 - \frac{\sigma_{\mathrm{afil}}}{\sigma_{\mathrm{orig}}}. \tag{6.9}$$

The noise reduction rate alone does, however, not consider the change in resolution. Therefore, a new figure of merit, the SNR-gain is introduced here. It sets into relation the standard deviation of noise in the adaptively filtered and linearly filtered image:

$$\mathrm{SNRG} = 1 - \frac{\sigma_{\mathrm{afil}}}{\sigma_{\mathrm{lfil}}}. \tag{6.10}$$

Both quantities are again evaluated for the 12 ROIs separately. The mean and standard deviation of both quantities over the different image regions are then computed. The mean values of the two quantities together can be interpreted as following:

- NNR and SNRG are approximately the same: This means that the adaptive filter has caused nearly no smoothing at the edge. Consequently, the MTF measured in the original and adaptively filtered images are nearly equivalent and the resulting linear filter has nearly no effect being applied to the noisy image. The NRR thus reflects the real gain in SNR.

- NRR is larger than the SNRG: This is the usual case if the edge was not perfectly preserved. If the edge got smoothed, the MTF from the adaptively filtered image falls below the original MTF. The resulting linear filter leading to the same average smoothing at the edge is a lowpass or bandpass filter. The linearly filtered image shows a reduced noise level, too. The real gain of the adaptive filter compared to the linear filter is thus given by the SNRG.

Further, the standard deviations of both quantities show how much variation in the achieved noise reduction and SNR-gain is obtained. If a high noise reduction rate is achieved in average, but a high variation between the different regions is present, this shows that the method works fine in some regions, but bad in other regions. This is a clear hint that the noise reduction method does not adapt to the local noise properties.

This evaluation strategy is now used for comparing different configurations of the presented noise reduction method in 2-D and 3-D. A comparison of the MTFs computed for the four examples presented in Fig. 6.2 is shown in Fig. 6.3. The MTF in the original noise-free image is compared to the MTFs computed from filtered images. Adaptive filters lead to different amounts of smoothing for different contrast-to-noise ratios at the edge of the circular object. Therefore, the MTFs are plotted for the different contrasts (1000, 100, 60 and 20 HU). Additionally, the MTFs resulting from only keeping the lowpass filtered approximation coefficients at the maximum decomposition level l_{max} and setting all detail coefficients to zero is shown. This gives the lower limit the MTF may reach if no structure

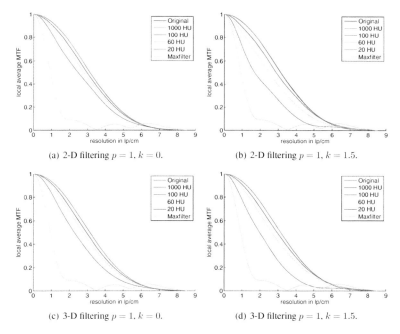

(a) 2-D filtering $p = 1, k = 0$.

(b) 2-D filtering $p = 1, k = 1.5$.

(c) 3-D filtering $p = 1, k = 0$.

(d) 3-D filtering $p = 1, k = 1.5$.

Figure 6.3: Local average MTF computed at the circular inlay of the elliptical phantom for different contrasts at the edge. Comparison of four configurations of the proposed filter in 2-D and 3-D.

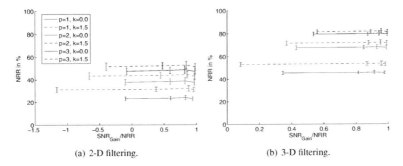

(a) 2-D filtering.   (b) 3-D filtering.

Figure 6.4: Noise-resolution-tradeoff - Comparison of NRR for different values of p with ($k = 1.5$) and without ($k = 0.0$) significance weights in 2-D and 3-D.

was detected and all computed weights were zero and is thus denoted as maxfilter in the following.

The MTFs in figure Fig. 6.3 show that for high CNR at the edge of the cylinder, the edge can be preserved perfectly. With decreasing CNR the edge preservation is reduced and the edges get smoothed. It is, however, noticeable that even in case of a CNR of 1, which corresponds to the contrast of 20 HU at the edge, the MTF is still much better than the MTF of the maxfilter. Of course, with increasing strength of the applied filtering, e. g. with increasing k the ability to detect low contrast edges also reduces. Consequently, the MTF decreases more drastically for low contrasts, if k is increased. Comparing the results of the 2-D and 3-D filtering, it can be seen that for higher contrasts a better edge preservation is achieved. For very low contrasts, like here the case of 20 HU, the smoothing at the edge is even slightly increased. As already mentioned above, it is however important to look at the noise-resolution-tradeoff and not just at noise or resolution separately. Therefore, the NRR is plotted against SNRG/NRR in Fig. 6.4. The performance of a noise reduction method is better the higher the NRR and the closer the ratio between SNRG and NRR is to 1. If the ratio between SNRG and NRR rate is 1, the edge was perfectly preserved and the complete NRR can be counted as a gain. In reality, however, this ratio falls below 1 if the edge was not perfectly preserved, e. g. for a lower CNR at the edge. This ratio can even become negative, if the linear filter, reaching the same average smoothing at the edge, leads to a overall stronger smoothing in the homogeneous image regions than the noise adaptive filter. In Fig. 6.4 each line represents a single configuration of the noise reduction method, where the four points of the line show the results achieved for the different CNR levels that were tested at the edge.

In Fig. 6.4 the noise-resolution-tradeoff is compared for different values of p with ($k = 1.5$) and without ($k = 0$) significance weighting in 2-D and 3-D. First of all it can be seen that with increasing p a stronger noise reduction can be achieved. If the significance weights are additionally used for the weighting of the coefficients, a higher noise reduction can be achieved for the same p. It is, however, noticeable that for low CNR the significance weights lead to increased smoothing at the edges. For higher contrasts at the edges, the significance weights show no negative influence on the resolution, just a positive effect on the noise reduction. In all cases it is noticeable, by comparing Fig. 6.4(a) and Fig. 6.4(b) that much better results with respect to noise reduction and edge preservation can be achieved in 3-D.

6.4.2   Example Images

In Fig. 6.5 an example slice, taken from a thoracic scan, is shown. The original slice (Fig. 6.5(a)) as well as the difference between the separate reconstructions (Fig. 6.5(b)) show directed noise due to high attenuation along the horizontal direction. An edge-detection is performed by correlation analysis between the approximation images, as can be seen in the weighting image at the first decomposition level in Fig. 6.5(e). In Fig. 6.5(f)-6.5(h) the combinations of correlation based weight and orientation dependent significance weights are shown for the horizontal, vertical and diagonal directions. This combination allows an adaptive, anisotropic denoising. The noise suppressed result image (3 levels of 2-D-Haar-DWT, denoised with $p = 1.0, k = 1.5$) is shown in Fig. 6.5(c), together with the difference to the original in Fig. 6.5(d). It can be seen that directed noise is reduced also in regions close to edges without noticeably affecting image resolution.

In Fig. 6.6 results are presented for a thin reconstructed slice (0.8 mm) taken from a CTA of a liver (see also difference images). The original noisy slice is shown in Fig. 6.6(a). In Fig. 6.6(c) the denoising result of the proposed method in 2-D is presented ($p = 1.0, k = 1.5$). Noticeably, the method adapts itself to the noise power in the image and removes noise more uniformly. In average, a reduction of pixel noise (standard deviation of noise in homogeneous region) of approximately 45% was achieved in 2-D. Nevertheless, the over-all image appearance is not very natural with respect to the residual noise power spectrum. The reason for this is that we used only a small neighborhood of 5×5 pixels for corre-lation computation. Therefore, the correlation analysis is not very reliable and some false correlations lead to noise remaining in the image. In comparison, the denoising in 3-D with $5 \times 5 \times 5$ neighborhoods and same parameter settings, shown in Fig. 6.6(e), is more effective. Noise is removed very well (up to 60%) in homogeneous areas and also close to edges. Even at lower contrasts, edges are still preserved. For example, the contrasted vessels in the liver are better visible in the noise suppressed image in comparison to the original.

6.5   Conclusions

In this chapter the combination of the two previously introduced wavelet based noise re-duction methods was presented. The correlation analysis between approximation coeffi-cients of the wavelet representation of two images was combined with an orientation and frequency dependent noise estimation. In addition to the correlation based weight, sig-nificance weights were introduced, which suppress coefficients in dependence on the esti-mated noise level of the wavelet coefficient. By combining the correlation and significance weight, the wavelet coefficients are treated differently not only depending on their posi-tion and the respective frequency band, but also for the different orientations. The result is that an anisotropic noise suppression becomes possible, which automatically adapts to the locally varying noise power. The anisotropic behavior is especially beneficial for datasets with directed noise, like in the hips or shoulder. Furthermore, the filtering approach was

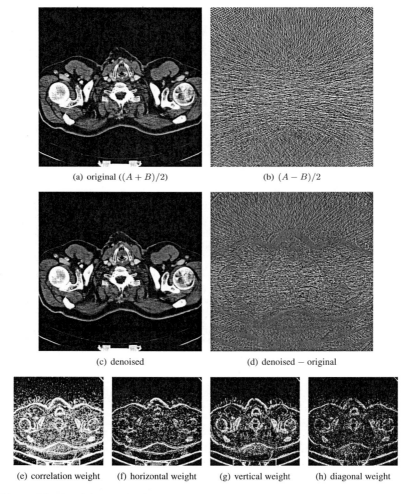

Figure 6.5: Denoising results for a thoracic slice, displayed with $c = 50$ and $w = 400$. Difference images are displayed with $c = 0$ and $w = 100$. The corresponding correlation based weight and the combinations with orientation dependent significance weights are shown for the first decomposition level (0 corresponds to black, 1 corresponds to white).

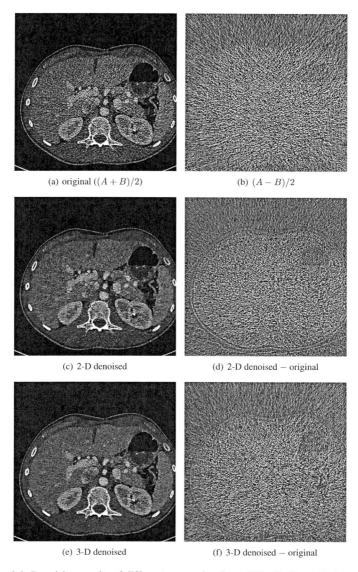

(a) original $((A + B)/2)$

(b) $(A - B)/2$

(c) 2-D denoised

(d) 2-D denoised − original

(e) 3-D denoised

(f) 3-D denoised − original

Figure 6.6: Denoising results of different approaches for a CTA of a liver, displayed with $c = 200$ and $w = 700$. The corresponding difference images are displayed with $c = 0$ and $w = 200$.

extended to 3-D. The application of the proposed method in 3-D showed higher noise reduction, up to 60%, and even improved edge-preservation.

Chapter 7

Noise Propagation Through Indirect Fan-Beam FPB Reconstruction

In CT, post-processing techniques are often applied to the reconstructed images. Depending on the application, which can vary from diagnostic tasks to treatment assessment problems, these techniques include, for example, edge-preserving filtering segmentation or image registration. It is a known fact that most standard post-processing techniques require a model for the noise in the reconstructed images. Frequently, a white Gaussian noise model based on a single, coarsely estimated parameter is assumed for the images. However, such a choice is suboptimal because the noise in CT images is non-stationary and object dependent. This chapter focuses on the problem of estimating the local noise variance in CT images. Having access to the image variance offers the potential to significantly improve the performance and outcome of post-processing techniques, as it has already been discussed in Chapter 5 and Chapter 6. For instance, it has been shown that taking into account the local noise variance for wavelet denoising [Bors 08d] or diffusion filtering [Maye 07] of CT reconstructions improves the noise suppression and gives more homogeneous results over the whole image domain.

The noise estimation in [Bors 08d] and [Maye 07] is obtained by dividing the measurements into two complete subsets yielding two images that are nearly independent in terms of noise, as it has been discussed in detail in Chapter 5 and Chapter 6. The experiments, however, showed that such an approach does not provide very reliable noise estimates. Also, the averaging step makes the variance estimates fairly non-local, whereas pixelwise estimates are desired.

A review of the literature shows that the image variance should preferably be computed using the knowledge that the noise in each individual image pixel is a direct result from the noise in the projections. In other words, the image variance can be obtained by propagating the noise in the data through the reconstruction pipeline. Such an approach is described in [Kak 01, Buzu 04] for FBP reconstruction from parallel-beam data, as it has been briefly summarized in Section 2.4.2. It is also used in [Pan 99, Pan 03, Wang 05, Wund 08] for direct fan-beam FBP reconstruction. All these references assume that the measurements are uncorrelated and that their variance is known. Moreover, they do not consider parallel-beam FBP reconstructions applied to rebinned fan-beam data. Reordering to parallel-beam projections is favored by many CT manufacturers for reasons of computational efficiency

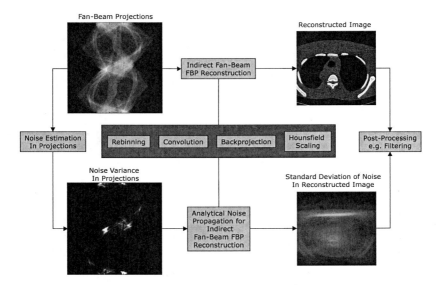

Figure 7.1: Overview of noise propagation method.

and ease in handling special scanning features such as the quarter-detector offset or redundant data.

The main contribution of this chapter, which has partially been published in [Bors 08a] can be summarized as follows: In this chapter a new method for the computation of the image variance in indirect fan-beam FBP reconstructions is introduced, where the data is first rebinned to parallel-beam geometry. The method follows the noise propagation scheme discussed above but has to deal with the difficulty that the rebinning step correlates the measurements together. To propagate the noise from one reconstruction step to the next, a modular technique is introduced that relies on results of linear system theory to compute any covariance terms that result from these steps. This technique makes the proposed method approximate but allows an easy implementation and efficient computations. Regarding the noise in the measurements, we also assume that noise is uncorrelated, as in [Kak 01, Buzu 04, Pan 99, Pan 03, Wang 05, Wund 08]. The proposed methodology is validated with three different phantoms, using computer-simulated data of known variance. Given that the ultimate goal is to obtain the image variance map in addition to the reconstruction, the statistical error in image variance calculation that results from estimating the variance in the data from a single measurement is additionally evaluated based on simulated and real data.

7.1 Methodology Overview

An overview of the here presented approach can be seen in Fig. 7.1. In addition to the reconstructed CT image, an estimate of the pixel-wise error should be computed. The local noise estimate can then be used for several post-processing methods that are performed on the reconstructed CT image. Noise reduction methods can, for example, be adapted to the local noise statistics.

Every step of the reconstruction pipeline needs to be modified in order to reconstruct noise variances. Starting with the noise estimates in the fan-beam projections, the noise variance and correlation are subsequently propagated from step to step through the reconstruction pipeline that is structured as follows:

- Rebinning from fan-beam projections to equidistantly spaced parallel projections.

- Convolution of the rebinned projections with the reconstruction kernel.

- Backprojection of the filtered projections.

- Hounsfield-scaling of reconstructed attenuation coefficients to normalized CT-values.

A detailed description of the reconstruction method can be found in Section 2.2.2. We rely strongly on the fact that all individual steps of the reconstruction pipeline (interpolations, convolution and backprojection) can be expressed as a linear combination of noisy data or random variables. For the variance of a linear combination of random variables taken from the random signal $x(t)$ the following holds [Weis]:

$$\text{Var}\left(\sum_i a_i x(t_i)\right) = \sum_i a_i^2 \text{Var}(x(t_i)) + \sum_i \sum_{j \neq i} a_i a_j \text{Cov}(x(t_i), x(t_j)), \qquad (7.1)$$

with a_i defining the weights, e.g., taken from a finite impulse response (FIR) filter. As can be seen from Eq. (7.1), in addition to the local variances $\text{Var}(x(t_i))$, the covariances $\text{Cov}(x(t_i), x(t_j))$ are needed to compute the noise variance of the linear combination of random variables. Additionally, for the exact computation of the noise variance after applying several linear filters in series, the propagation of the covariance matrix from step to step would be needed. This makes the whole processing complicated and often computationally inefficient. Here, an original approximate method is proposed that estimates the covariance terms based on linear system theory.

When the variances, $\text{Var}(x(t))$, are available, it is known that the covariance between the values of the random signal $x(t)$ at two positions t_1 and t_2 can be computed using the autocorrelation coefficient function (ACCF) $\rho_{xx}(t_1, t_2)$ and the local variances, as

$$\text{Cov}(x(t_1), x(t_2)) = \sqrt{\text{Var}(x(t_1))\text{Var}(x(t_2))}\rho_{xx}(t_1, t_2). \qquad (7.2)$$

However, the above equation still does not facilitate the model and implementation because it requires the computation of the local autocorrelation coefficients. The propagation of the variances and correlations from step to step would be much easier and could be performed using linear system theory if wide-sense stationary (WSS) signals could be assumed. The requirement for wide-sense stationarity is that the mean and autocorrelation are shift-invariant. In CT projections, noise is additive and can be assumed to be zero-mean. Hence the assumption that the mean is shift-invariant is fulfilled. If the correlation lengths are small and the linear combinations are only performed on coefficients concentrated around a given sample, it is a good approximation to assume that the ACCF is shift-invariant. In the following the random signal at any step is assumed to be a WSS signal in the sense that the ACCF can be estimated as a function of the parameter $\tau = t_2 - t_1$. Eq. (7.2) can then be rewritten as

$$\text{Cov}(x(t_1), x(t_2)) = \sqrt{\text{Var}(x(t_1))\text{Var}(x(t_2))}\rho_{xx}(\tau). \tag{7.3}$$

The ACCF can be expressed as the normalized autocorrelation function:

$$\rho_{xx}(\tau) = \varphi_{xx}(\tau)/\varphi_{xx}(0), \tag{7.4}$$

where the autocorrelation function (ACF), $\varphi_{xx}(\tau)$, of a zero-mean WSS signal is:

$$\varphi_{xx}(\tau) = \varphi_{xx}(t_1, t_1 + \tau) = \varphi_{xx}(t_1, t_2) = \mathcal{E}\{x(t_1)x(t_2)\}. \tag{7.5}$$

In the ideal case of perfectly uncorrelated data, the ACCF is just a delta function, which is zero everywhere except for $\tau = 0$. The application of a linear shift-invariant filter $h(t)$ to a random signal $x(t)$ changes its autocorrelation and thus also its autocorrelation coefficient function. Even if a perfectly uncorrelated signal is the input to a pipeline of several linear operations, the outputs at the intermediate steps are no longer perfectly uncorrelated. Therefore, the amount of correlation after performing a linear operation needs to be modeled as well. The response of linear shift-invariant (LSI) system to the random signal $x(t)$ is computed by convolution:

$$y(t) = x(t) * h(t). \tag{7.6}$$

The output signal $y(t)$ is still a random process. For the mean of the output signal $y(t)$ the following holds:

$$\mu_y(t) = \mathcal{E}\{y(t)\} = \mathcal{E}\{x(t)\} * h(t) = \mu_x(t) * h(t), \tag{7.7}$$

where $\mu_x(t)$ is the mean of the input. Consequently, filtering a zero-mean signal results in zero-mean output. If the input signal $x(t)$ is a WSS signal, then the autocorrelation function of the output $y(t)$ also only depends on τ and can be written as [Oppe 96, Giro 01]:

$$\varphi_{yy}(\tau) = \varphi_{xx}(\tau) * \varphi_{hh}(\tau). \tag{7.8}$$

This means the ACF of the output signal can be computed by convolving the ACF of the input signal with the ACF of the filter. The ACF of the filter is given as [Oppe 96, Giro 01]:

$$\varphi_{hh}(\tau) = h(\tau) * h^*(-\tau), \tag{7.9}$$

where $h^*(\tau)$ is the complex conjugate of $h(\tau)$. The ACCF, as defined in Eq. (7.4), is just a normalized version of the ACF. Thus, it is valid to directly convolve the ACCF of the input, $\rho_{xx}(\tau)$, with the filter ACCF, $\rho_{hh}(\tau)$, to compute the ACCF at the output:

$$\rho_{yy}(\tau) = \frac{\tilde{\rho}_{yy}(\tau)}{\tilde{\rho}_{yy}(0)}, \quad \text{with} \quad \tilde{\rho}_{yy}(\tau) = \rho_{xx}(\tau) * \rho_{hh}(\tau). \tag{7.10}$$

The methodology used for noise propagation can be summarized as following: In order to compute a pixel-wise estimate of the noise variance in the reconstructed image, the noise variance estimates and the correlation within the data is propagated from step to step through the reconstruction pipeline. The starting point of the noise propagation method is an estimate of the noise variance and noise correlation in the acquired fan-beam projections. For simplicity, we assume here that noise in the fan-beam projections is perfectly uncorrelated, which is valid as long as crosstalk at the detector, afterglow and tube-current variations are negligibly small. Consequently, the ACCF of the noise in the fan-beam projections is assumed to be a delta function. For each stage of the reconstruction pipeline the variance and ACCF are updated as follows:

1. The variance of the linear combination of random variables is computed according to Eq. (7.1). The covariances needed for Eq. (7.1) are approximated using the ACCF and the local variances of the input to the current stage of the pipeline, as described in Eq. (7.3). Note again that only the ACCF is modeled under a wide-sense stationarity assumption. By using the local variances for the computation, the non-stationarity of noise is taken into account.

2. The current pipeline stage changes the correlation within the data. Therefore, the ACCF that is used for the next processing step needs to be updated. This is done by modeling interpolation and filtering steps to be represented by a linear shift-invariant filter. The ACCF corresponding to the output of the filtered signal is computed according to Eq. (7.10).

7.2 Noise Propagation Through Indirect Fan-Beam FBP Reconstruction

The estimates of the noise variances in the fan-beam projections are the input to the algorithm for noise propagation. These estimates can be based either on repeated measurements of the same object, or just one single measurement and a calibrated noise model. In the following, a detailed description is presented, on how the above introduced methodology can be applied to all single steps of the reconstruction pipeline.

7.2.1 Rebinning

Starting with the noise variances, $\mathrm{Var}(P_{\mathrm{k,l}}^{\mathrm{fan}})$, and ACCF, $\rho^{\mathrm{fan}}(\alpha, \beta)$, of the acquired fan-beam projections, the first step of the reconstruction pipeline is the rebinning to parallel-beam projections. First, during azimuthal rebinning, Eq. (2.10) is applied to obtain hybrid projections depending on the parallel projection angle θ and the fan angle β. For interpolating the noise variances Eq. (7.1) is applied to Eq. (2.10), giving:

$$\mathrm{Var}(P_{\mathrm{m,l}}^{\mathrm{hyb}}) = \sum_{k=1}^{N_{2\pi f}} (h^{\mathrm{azi}}(\tilde{\alpha}_{\mathrm{m,l}} - \alpha_k))^2 \mathrm{Var}(P_{\mathrm{k,l}}^{\mathrm{fan}}) +$$

$$\sum_{k=1}^{N_{2\pi f}} \sum_{\substack{\tilde{k}=1 \\ \tilde{k} \neq k}}^{N_{2\pi f}} h^{\mathrm{azi}}(\tilde{\alpha}_{\mathrm{m,l}} - \alpha_k) h^{\mathrm{azi}}(\tilde{\alpha}_{\mathrm{m,l}} - \alpha_{\tilde{k}}) \mathrm{Cov}(P_{\mathrm{k,l}}^{\mathrm{fan}}, P_{\tilde{k},l}^{\mathrm{fan}}). \quad (7.11)$$

The covariances are computed based on Eq. (7.3) as

$$\text{Cov}(P_{k,l}^{\text{fan}}, P_{\bar{k},l}^{\text{fan}}) = \sqrt{\text{Var}(P_{k,l}^{\text{fan}})\text{Var}(P_{\bar{k},l}^{\text{fan}})}\rho^{\text{fan}}(\alpha_k - \alpha_{\bar{k}}, 0) \tag{7.12}$$

As already mentioned before, noise in the fan-beam projections is assumed to be perfectly uncorrelated. Thus, the ACCF of noise in the fan-beam projections is a delta function, i.e. $\rho^{\text{fan}}(\alpha_k - \alpha_{\bar{k}}, \beta_l - \beta_l) = \rho^{\text{fan}}(\alpha_k - \alpha_{\bar{k}}, 0) = 0$. Consequently, the covariances in Eq. (7.11) are all zero.

After that the complementary rebinning is performed. Two different cases need to be distinguished here, too. If the quarter-detector-offset is used, two projections with an offset of π are interleaved in order to increase the resolution within one projection. This step does not influence the single variance values. They are also just interleaved:

$$\text{Var}(P_{i,2l-1}^{\text{com}}) = \text{Var}(P_{i,l}^{\text{hyb}}), \quad \text{and} \quad \text{Var}(P_{i,2l}^{\text{com}}) = \text{Var}(P_{i+N_{\pi p}, N_p+1-l}^{\text{hyb}}). \tag{7.13}$$

If no quarter detector offset is used, redundant measurements are averaged together. For the variances again Eq. (7.1) is applied:

$$\text{Var}(P_{i,l}^{\text{com}}) = \frac{1}{4}\left(\text{Var}(P_{i,l}^{\text{hyb}}) + \text{Var}(P_{i+N_{\pi p}, N_p+1-l}^{\text{hyb}})\right) + \frac{1}{2}\text{Cov}(P_{i,l}^{\text{hyb}}, P_{i+N_{\pi p}, N_p+1-l}^{\text{hyb}}). \tag{7.14}$$

The covariances again cancel out if noise in the fan-beam data is assumed to be uncorrelated. The azimuthal and complementary interpolations do not introduce correlations to the hybrid projections in β direction. Thus, for the last rebinning step the data can still be assumed to be uncorrelated. After this interpolation the corresponding noise variances $\text{Var}(P(\theta, t))$ for every discrete parallel projection is obtained by:

$$\text{Var}(P_{i,n}^{\text{par}}) = \sum_{j=1}^{N_c}(h^{\text{rad}}(\tilde{\beta}_n - \beta_j'))^2\text{Var}(P_{i,j}^{\text{com}}) +$$

$$\sum_{j=1}^{N_c}\sum_{\substack{j=1 \\ j\neq j}}^{N_c} h^{\text{rad}}(\tilde{\beta}_n - \beta_j')h^{\text{rad}}(\tilde{\beta}_n - \beta_j')\text{Cov}(P_{i,j}^{\text{com}}, P_{i,j}^{\text{com}}). \tag{7.15}$$

With the same reasoning as above, the covariances are zero, if uncorrelated fan-beam projections are assumed.

After rebinning, noise in the parallel projections and between neighboring views is no longer uncorrelated. The interpolation filter function used for azimuthal rebinning is denoted as h^{azi} and the radial interpolation filter is h^{rad}. Based on these two filters the autocorrelation coefficient function is computed that describes the amount of correlation introduced to the data during the rebinning process. The complete interpolation filter is modeled as a separable 2-D-filter:

$$h^{\text{ipol}}(\theta, t) = h^{\text{azi}}(\theta) \cdot h^{\text{rad}}(t), \tag{7.16}$$

which is an approximation since the (θ, t)-coordinates are not orthogonal relative to the (α, β)-coordinates. Therefore, the ACCF $\rho^{ipol}(t)$ corresponding to the 2-D interpolation filter is:

$$\rho^{ipol}(\theta, t) = h(\theta, t)/h(0, 0), \quad h(\theta, t) = h^{\text{ipol}}(\theta, t) * *h^{\text{ipol}}(\theta, t), \tag{7.17}$$

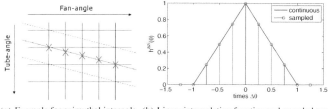

(a) Example for azimuthal interpola- (b) Linear interpolation function and sampled ver-
tion.   sion

Figure 7.2: Example for linear interpolation weights appearing during azimuthal rebinning. The continuous interpolation function is sampled only at few positions.

where $**$ denotes a 2-D convolution. Because of the assumption of perfectly uncorrelated noise in the fan-beam projections, the updated ACCF after rebinning is equivalent to $\rho^{rpol}(t)$. The convolution according to Eq. (7.10) with the ACCF of the fan-beam projections, which is a delta function, has no effect.

The approximation of the correlation introduced to the data during rebinning by the continuous interpolation functions, as described above, is not the best solution when working with discrete data. The resampling during azimuthal interpolation usually leads to a very regular interpolation pattern, as illustrated in Fig. 7.2(a). Therefore, the interpolation function is repeatedly evaluated at few positions only. Depending on how the two grids lie to each other the continuous approximation might under- or overestimate the correlation within the data. The continuous case assumes that all positions between the discrete grid points are interpolated with the same frequency, which is not the case during the rebinning procedure described above. The problem can be easily understood regarding one simple example. If linear interpolation is used for computing samples that are placed perfectly in the center between the original samples, the maximum of correlation is introduced to the data. Two neighboring samples were computed by one half from the same original noisy data placed between them. The other extreme would be that both grids are perfectly lying on each other. Then no further correlation is introduced to the data at all. This example already shows the importance of taking into account the discrete sampling of the data.

The average functions corresponding to the sampled azimuthal and radial interpolation functions are computed taking into account the weights that really appear during interpolation, which is basically a sampled version of the continuous interpolation function, as shown in Fig. 7.2(b). The function corresponding to the azimuthal rebinning is computed as:

$$\tilde{h}^{azi}(\theta) = \sum_{m=1}^{N_{2\pi p}} \sum_{l=1}^{N_f} \sum_{k=1}^{N_{2\pi f}} h^{azi}(\theta)\delta(\theta - \frac{\tilde{\alpha}_{m,l} + \alpha_k}{\Delta\alpha}\Delta\theta). \tag{7.18}$$

During radial rebinning an interpolation from a non-uniform to a uniform grid is performed. This means that the distances between neighboring samples varies within a projection. The relative distance between neighboring samples within a projection is plotted in Fig. 7.3(a). This has the effect that interpolation weights are not used with the same frequency, as can be seen in Fig. 7.3(c). The distribution of linear interpolation weights depends on the channel number, as shown in Fig. 7.3(b). From this plot it can be seen

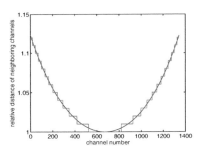

(a) Relative sampling distance between neighboring channels

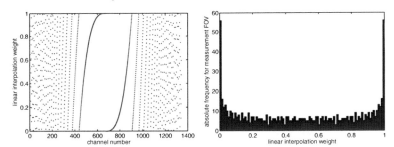

(b) Linear interpolation weights for different channels

(c) Histogram of linear interpolation weights for measurement FOV

Figure 7.3: Example for linear interpolation weights appearing during radial rebinning.

quite clearly that close to the center ray the two grids are more or less lying onto each other, because weights close to 0 and 1 appear. At the outer borders the weights seem to be more randomly arranged. In practice this means that for reconstructions within a small FOV around the iso-center nearly no correlations are introduced to the data during radial rebinning. If a large FOV is reconstructed, the outer rays are needed for the reconstruction, too. Thus stronger correlated data is used. This should be taken into account in estimating the amount of correlation within the data after rebinning. One approach is to compute the average sampled interpolation function that corresponds to radial rebinning. Here, only those channels ($n \in [n_{min}, n_{max}]$) within the projection are taken into account that are used for the reconstruction of the current FOV:

$$\tilde{h}^{\mathrm{rad}}(t) = \sum_{n=n_{min}}^{n_{max}} \sum_{j=1}^{N_c} h^{\mathrm{rad}}(t)\delta(t - \tilde{\beta}_n + \beta'_j). \tag{7.19}$$

Instead of working with the real continuous interpolation functions, the averaged sampled versions presented in Eq. (7.18) and Eq. (7.19) are used instead in Eq. (7.16).

7.2.2 Convolution

The next step in the reconstruction pipeline is the convolution of the parallel projections $P(\theta, t)$ with the kernel function $k(t)$ along the row direction t, as described in Eq. (2.18). The noise variance in the filtered projections $\mathrm{Var}(P(\theta, t))$ can thus be computed based on Eq. (7.1).

Basically, the noise propagation through the convolution can be split into two parts: the convolution with the squared filtering kernel and the consideration of the covariances. The convolution of the noise variances in the parallel projections with the squared filtering kernel has also been considered in the theoretical analysis presented in [Buzu 04] and [Kak 01]. However, the experiments will show that the covariance terms of the data within the same projections are essential for getting reliable noise estimates. Altogether, the noise variance in the filtered projections can be computed according to:

$$\mathrm{Var}(P_{i,n}^{\mathrm{fil}}) = \Delta t^2 \left(\sum_{s=1}^{N_p} P_{i,s}^{\mathrm{par}} k^2(t_n - t_s) + \sum_{s=1}^{N_p} \sum_{\substack{r=1 \\ r \neq s}}^{N_p} \mathrm{Cov}(P_{i,s}^{\mathrm{par}}, P_{i,r}^{\mathrm{par}}) k(t_n - t_s) k(t_n - t_r) \right). \tag{7.20}$$

The covariance between two channels within one parallel projection can be approximated using the autocorrelation coefficient function in Eq. (7.17):

$$\mathrm{Cov}(P_{i,s}^{\mathrm{par}}, P_{i,r}^{\mathrm{par}}) \approx \sqrt{\mathrm{Var}(P_{i,s}^{\mathrm{par}})\mathrm{Var}(P_{i,r}^{\mathrm{par}})}\rho^{\mathrm{ipol}}(0, t_s - t_r). \tag{7.21}$$

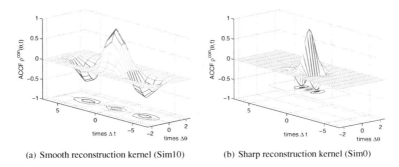

(a) Smooth reconstruction kernel (Sim10)   (b) Sharp reconstruction kernel (Sim0)

Figure 7.4: Autocorrelation coefficient functions after convolution for two different reconstruction kernels.

The projections are sampled with the sampling distance Δt. Consequently, Eq. (7.21) can be reformulated such that the distance between t_s and t_r in discrete steps of size Δt is included:

$$\text{Var}(P_{i,n}^{\text{fil}}) = \Delta t^2 \left(\sum_{s=1}^{N_p} k^2(t_n - t_s) P_{i,s}^{\text{par}} + \sum_{q=1}^{q_{\text{max}}} \rho^{ipol}(0, q\Delta t) \times \right.$$
$$\sum_{s=1}^{N_p} \left(\sqrt{\text{Var}(P_{i,s}^{\text{par}})\text{Var}(P_{i,s+q}^{\text{par}})} k(t_n - t_s)k(t_n - t_s - q\Delta t) + \right.$$
$$\left. \left. \sqrt{\text{Var}(P_{i,s}^{\text{par}})\text{Var}(P_{i,s-q}^{\text{par}})} k(t_n - t_s)k(t_n - t_s + q\Delta t) \right) \right). \quad (7.22)$$

The covariance parts are consequently implemented by additional convolutions. The parameter q_{max} controls how many neighboring channels are taken into account for covariance computation. Usually, the autocorrelation function $\rho^{ipol}(\theta, t)$ very rapidly goes to zero. This means that only channels in a small neighborhood are correlated. Therefore, the maximum distance between the channels that need to be considered and thus q_{max} can be chosen in dependence of the ACCF:

$$q_{\text{max}} = \text{argmax}_{q \in \mathbb{N}} \left\{ \rho^{ipol}(0, q\Delta t) > \epsilon \right\}. \quad (7.23)$$

Those q for which the correlation coefficient at $q\Delta t$ is below a certain small threshold ϵ are neglected in Eq. (7.22). Typical values for ϵ are in the range of 0.01.

The convolution process inside the reconstruction pipeline introduces further correlations within the parallel projections. In order to model this for the next step, the ACCF after filtering needs to be computed. The filter ACCF is computed based on Eq. (7.4) and Eq. (7.9) as

$$\rho_{kk}(t) = \frac{\varphi_{kk}(t)}{\varphi_{kk}(0)} \quad \text{with} \quad \varphi_{kk}(t) = k(t) * k^*(-t). \quad (7.24)$$

The correlation inside the data after convolution is described by convolution of the ACCF after rebinning with the filter ACCF along the direction of t followed by normalization, as described in Eq. (7.10):

$$\rho^{con}(\theta, t) = \frac{\tilde{\rho}^{con}(\theta, t)}{\tilde{\rho}^{con}(0,0)}, \quad \tilde{\rho}^{con}(\theta, t) = \rho^{ipol}(\theta, t) * \rho_{kk}(t). \tag{7.25}$$

Two examples for different convolution kernels are shown in Fig. 7.4.

7.2.3 Backprojection

After the filtering with the convolution kernel the next step in the reconstruction pipeline is the backprojection into image plane. For each image pixel $\mathbf{x}$ the sum over all $N_{\pi p}$ parallel projection angles $\theta \in [0, \pi[$ is computed according to Eq. (2.20). The noise variance of the reconstructed attenuation coefficients $\mathrm{Var}(\mu(\mathbf{x}))$ then amounts to:

$$\mathrm{Var}(\mu(\mathbf{x})) = \Delta\theta^2 \left(\sum_{i=1}^{N_{\pi p}} \mathrm{Var}(P_i^{fil}(\mathbf{x})) + \sum_{i=1}^{N_{\pi p}} \sum_{\substack{j=1 \\ j \neq i}}^{N_{\pi p}} \mathrm{Cov}(P_i^{fil}(\mathbf{x}), P_j^{fil}(\mathbf{x})) \right) \approx$$

$$\approx \Delta\theta^2 \left(\sum_{i=1}^{N_{\pi p}} \mathrm{Var}(P_i^{fil}(\mathbf{x})) + \sum_{i=1}^{N_{\pi p}} \sum_{j=1}^{j_{max}} \left(\mathrm{Cov}(P_i^{fil}(\mathbf{x}), P_{i+j}^{fil}(\mathbf{x})) + \mathrm{Cov}(P_i^{fil}(\mathbf{x}), P_{i-j}^{fil}(\mathbf{x})) \right) \right). \tag{7.26}$$

During the reconstruction algorithm only the azimuthal rebinning introduces a correlation between directly neighboring projections. Thus, only the covariances between few neighboring projections need to be taken into account. It is again possible to determine j_{max} based on the ACCF after convolution in direction of θ:

$$j_{max} = \mathrm{argmax}_{j \in \mathbb{N}} \left\{ \rho^{con}(j\Delta\theta, 0) > \epsilon \right\}. \tag{7.27}$$

For getting the projection values $P_i^{fil}(\mathbf{x})$ an interpolation is necessary, as described in Eq. (2.21). Consequently, the covariances in Eq. (7.26) can be computed by:

$$\mathrm{Cov}(P_i^{fil}(\mathbf{x}), P_j^{fil}(\mathbf{x})) = \sum_{n=1}^{N_p} \sum_{m=1}^{N_p} h^{bpj}(\tilde{t}_i(\mathbf{x}) - t_n) h^{bpj}(\tilde{t}_j(\mathbf{x}) - t_m) \mathrm{Cov}(P_{i,n}^{fil}, P_{j,m}^{fil}), \tag{7.28}$$

with

$$\tilde{t}_i(\mathbf{x}) = x \sin\theta_i - y \cos\theta_i. \tag{7.29}$$

Accordingly, the variance can be computed as a special case by:

$$\mathrm{Var}(P_i^{fil}(\mathbf{x})) = \sum_{n=1}^{N_p} \left(h^{bpj}(\tilde{t}_i(\mathbf{x}) - t_n) \right)^2 \mathrm{Var}(P_{i,n}^{fil}) +$$

$$\sum_{n=1}^{N_p} \sum_{\substack{m=1 \\ m \neq n}}^{N_p} h^{bpj}(\tilde{t}_i(\mathbf{x}) - t_n) h^{bpj}(\tilde{t}_i(\mathbf{x}) - t_m) \mathrm{Cov}(P_{i,n}^{fil}, P_{i,m}^{fil}). \tag{7.30}$$

The covariances are approximated based on the ACCF given in Eq. (7.25):

$$\text{Cov}(P_{i,n}^{\text{fil}}, P_{j,m}^{\text{fil}}) \approx \sqrt{\text{Var}(P_{i,n}^{\text{fil}})\text{Var}(P_{j,m}^{\text{fil}})}\rho^{\text{con}}(\theta_i - \theta_j, t_n - t_m). \tag{7.31}$$

On the first glance, it seems that Eq. (7.28) and Eq. (7.30) require a large number of computations because of the included double sums. However, the interpolation functions are different from zero only for a few neighboring channels. If linear interpolation is used, as defined in Eq. (2.23), e.g. only two neighboring channels within one projection are considered and consequently, only four summands are required in Eq. (7.28).

7.2.4 Hounsfield Scaling

The reconstructed attenuation coefficients are usually normalized to Hounsfield-Units. This is done as described in Eq. (2.22). In order to estimate the noise in the normalized reconstructed data, the following equation needs to be used:

$$\text{Var}(f(\mathbf{x})) = \text{Var}(\mu(\mathbf{x}))\left(\frac{1000}{\mu_w}\right)^2 \text{HU}^2. \tag{7.32}$$

Consequently, the standard deviation of noise $\sigma(\mathbf{x})$ in the reconstructed and normalized image can be computed by

$$\sigma(\mathbf{x}) = \sqrt{\text{Var}(f(\mathbf{x}))}. \tag{7.33}$$

7.2.5 Covariance Between Reconstructed Hounsfield Values

The above presented theory can be extended to compute the covariance between reconstructed Hounsfield values. Therefore, the correlation between neighboring pixels can be determined analytically, too. The covariance between two normalized reconstructed pixel values at two arbitrary positions $\mathbf{x}_1$ and $\mathbf{x}_2$ can be computed as:

$$\text{Cov}(f(\mathbf{x}_1), f(\mathbf{x}_2)) = \left(\frac{1000}{\mu_w}\right)^2 \text{Cov}(\mu(\mathbf{x}_1), \mu(\mathbf{x}_2)) \text{ HU}^2. \tag{7.34}$$

This equation can be used for computing the complete covariance matrix of an image. According to the variance computation in Eq. (7.26), which is just a special case of the covariance, the covariance amounts to:

$$\text{Cov}(\mu(\mathbf{x}_1), \mu(\mathbf{x}_2)) = \Delta\theta^2 \sum_{i=1}^{N_{\pi p}} \sum_{j=1}^{N_{\pi p}} \text{Cov}(P_i^{\text{fil}}(\mathbf{x}_1), P_j^{\text{fil}}(\mathbf{x}_2)) \approx$$

$$\approx \Delta\theta^2 \sum_{i=1}^{N_{\pi p}} \sum_{j=-j_{max}}^{j_{max}} \text{Cov}(P_i^{\text{fil}}(\mathbf{x}_1), P_{i+j}^{\text{fil}}(\mathbf{x}_2)). \tag{7.35}$$

Here, again the approximation is used that only few neighboring projections are correlated because of the azimuthal rebinning. The number of neighboring projections is determined based on the ACCF as given in Eq. (7.27). The covariance between interpolated values taken out of two parallel projections is computed very similar to Eq. (7.28):

$$\text{Cov}(P_i^{\text{fil}}(\mathbf{x}_1), P_j^{\text{fil}}(\mathbf{x}_2)) = \sum_{n=1}^{N_p} \sum_{m=1}^{N_p} h^{\text{bpj}}(\tilde{t}_i(\mathbf{x}_1) - t_n) h^{\text{bpj}}(\tilde{t}_j(\mathbf{x}_2) - t_m) \text{Cov}(P_{i,n}^{\text{fil}}, P_{j,m}^{\text{fil}}),$$
(7.36)

where

$$\tilde{t}_i(\mathbf{x}_1) = x_1 \sin \theta_i - y_1 \cos \theta_i, \quad \text{and} \quad \tilde{t}_j(\mathbf{x}_2) = x_2 \sin \theta_j - y_2 \cos \theta_j.$$
(7.37)

Finally, the same approximation that is used for the variance computation can be applied here:

$$\text{Cov}(P_{i,n}^{\text{fil}}, P_{j,m}^{\text{fil}}) \approx \sqrt{\text{Var}(P_{i,n}^{\text{fil}}) \text{Var}(P_{j,m}^{\text{fil}})} \rho^{\text{con}}(\theta_i - \theta_j, t_n - t_m).$$
(7.38)

The correlation coefficient between two image pixels can then be computed using Eq. (7.34) and the local variances from Eq. (7.32):

$$\rho^{\text{img}}(\mathbf{x}_1, \mathbf{x}_2) = \frac{\text{Cov}(f(\mathbf{x}_1), f(\mathbf{x}_2))}{\sqrt{\text{Var}(f(\mathbf{x}_1)) \text{Var}(f(\mathbf{x}_2))}}.$$
(7.39)

7.3 Experimental Evaluation

The analytic model presented in the previous section makes use of some assumptions and approximations, leading to a systematic error of the method. In addition, the method uses noisy projection data as input to the noise estimation. This leads to an additional intrinsic statistical uncertainty. To quantify systematic and statistical uncertainty of the presented method, Monte-Carlo simulations were carried out.

7.3.1 Simulation

Three analytical phantoms were used for the evaluation of the noise propagation method:

- The FORBILD thorax phantom, in the following denoted as thorax phantom, is shown in Fig. 7.5(a). It is reconstructed at a FOV of 41 cm, the slice is positioned at $z = 0$ cm.

- A modified version of the FORBILD thorax phantom, in the following denoted as shoulder phantom, is shown in Fig. 7.5(d). It is reconstructed at a FOV of 51 cm, the slice is positioned at $z = 14$ cm. One of the lungs was translated 0.75 cm in z-direction in order to achieve more antisymmetry.

- The FORBILD head phantom with ears is shown in Fig. 7.5(g). It is reconstructed at a FOV of 25 cm, the slice is positioned at $z = 0$ cm.

For all three phantoms, noise-free fan-beam projections were simulated using 1160 projections, 672 detector channels and a quarter detector offset. The following physical parameters were selected for the simulation: focus width 0.7 mm, anode angle $-82°$, delta beta $\Delta\beta = 360/4640$ mm, 80 kV. The indirect fan-beam FBP reconstruction was performed in combination with four different reconstruction kernels. The MTFs of the kernels are displayed in Fig. 7.6. For the noise propagation method the parameter $\epsilon = 0.01$ was used in Eq. (7.23) and Eq. (7.27). The parameters q_{max} and j_{max} are thus equal to 1 for all experiments.

7.3.2   Accuracy of the Noise Propagation

CT-image noise estimates were built according to the following three procedures:

a) Noise free projections were used for a Poisson-distributed noise estimation. The propagation through the analytical model yields $\sigma_a(\mathbf{x})$.

b) Monte-Carlo simulations of $N_{MC} = 10000$ CT images were generated. For each image, Poisson-distributed noise was added to the projections. Pixel-wise noise computation from the N_{MC} reconstructed images gives $\sigma_b(\mathbf{x})$.

c) In parallel, for each of the N_{MC} images the noisy projections were used for Poisson-distributed noise estimation. The propagation through the analytical model yields $\sigma_c(\mathbf{x})$ and $Var(\sigma_c(\mathbf{x}))$.

Procedure a) provides the expectation value for the CT image noise according to the proposed method. The standard deviation computed in b) yields the gold standard to compare with. The standard deviation images $\sigma_a(\mathbf{x})$ and $\sigma_b(\mathbf{x})$ are used to determine the systematic error of the proposed method on a per-pixel basis. The pixelwise relative error is defined as:

$$r_\Delta(\mathbf{x}) = \frac{\sigma_a(\mathbf{x}) - \sigma_b(\mathbf{x})}{\sigma_b(\mathbf{x})}. \qquad (7.40)$$

The noise propagation method is precise if the relative pixelwise errors are small on the complete image domain. Therefore, the average relative error

$$\bar{r}_\Delta = \frac{1}{N} \sum_{i=1}^{N} r_\Delta(\mathbf{x}_i), \qquad (7.41)$$

and its variance

$$\sigma_{r_\Delta}^2 = \frac{1}{N-1} \sum_{i=1}^{N} (r_\Delta(\mathbf{x}_i) - \bar{r}_\Delta)^2, \qquad (7.42)$$

over the different image pixels is computed, where N is the number of image pixels and $r_\Delta(\mathbf{x}_i)$ is the relative error at pixel position $\mathbf{x}_i$. The average quadratic error, normalized on a per-pixel basis is defined as:

$$s_\Delta = \sqrt{\frac{1}{N} \sum_{i=1}^{N} (r_\Delta(\mathbf{x}_i))^2} = \sqrt{(\bar{r}_\Delta)^2 + \frac{N-1}{N}\sigma_{r_\Delta}^2}. \qquad (7.43)$$

Measuring the variance of the noise prediction during procedure c) exhibits its intrinsic statistical uncertainty for a given dose and object. The ultimate goal of the here presented noise propagation method is to get a variance map in addition to a reconstructed image, using one single measurement. Then the input to the noise propagation is no longer the exact noise variance in the projections, but a noisy estimate. Each of the $N_{MC} = 10000$

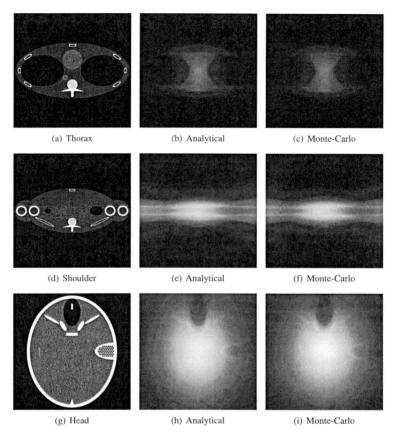

(a) Thorax   (b) Analytical   (c) Monte-Carlo

(d) Shoulder   (e) Analytical   (f) Monte-Carlo

(g) Head   (h) Analytical   (i) Monte-Carlo

Figure 7.5: Phantoms used for evaluation reconstructed with Sim50 (Thorax: 30 cm FOV, display: w=50, c=400, Shoulder: 51 cm FOV, display: w=50, c=900, Head: 25 cm FOV, display: w=50, c=900), together with analytical noise estimates and estimates from 10000 noisy realizations (Thorax noise display: w=25, c=50, Shoulder and Head noise display: w=50, c=150).

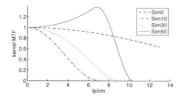

Figure 7.6: MTFs of kernels used for the experiments.

noisy projections are used for estimating the noise variance in the projections respectively and are then separately propagated through the reconstruction algorithm giving N_{MC} standard deviation images $\sigma_{c,m}(\mathbf{x})$ with $m = 1, ..., N_{MC}$. From the stack of standard deviation images the pixelwise mean $\bar{\sigma}_c(\mathbf{x})$ and variance $\text{Var}(\sigma_c(\mathbf{x}))$ can be computed as:

$$\bar{\sigma}_c(\mathbf{x}) = \frac{1}{N_{MC}} \sum_m \sigma_{c,m}(\mathbf{x}), \tag{7.44}$$

$$\text{Var}(\sigma_c(\mathbf{x})) = \frac{1}{N_{MC} - 1} \sum_m (\sigma_{c,m}(\mathbf{x}) - \bar{\sigma}_{c,m}(\mathbf{x}))^2. \tag{7.45}$$

The pixelwise standard deviation of the standard deviation images $\sigma(\sigma_c(\mathbf{x})) = \sqrt{\text{Var}(\sigma_c(\mathbf{x}))}$ is a measure for how stable the noise variances can be reproduced using different noise realizations. For all three phantoms the values in $\text{Var}(\sigma_c(\mathbf{x}))$ were well below 0.1%.

Table 7.1: Evaluation of the systematic error of the method proposed. Numbers are quoted in percent (%).

Thorax	Sim10	Sim30	Sim50	Sim0
$\bar{\sigma}_b$	3.7	5.8	13.2	10.2
$r_{\Delta,1}$	-22.3±8.5	-11.0±9.8	5.5±11.2	3.3±9.7
s_Δ	23.9	14.8	12.5	10.2
$r_{\Delta,2}$	-18.4±8.9	-8.0±10.1	5.8±11.2	3.7±9.7
s_Δ	20.4	12.9	12.6	10.4
$r_{\Delta,3}$	-16.4±7.4	-5.9±7.7	8.3±8.9	6.1±7.1
s_Δ	18.0	9.7	12.2	9.4
$r_{\Delta,4}$	-3.6±3.6	-1.6±3.3	1.2±2.4	0.7±2.2
s_Δ	5.3	3.9	2.8	2.3
Shoulder	Sim10	Sim30	Sim50	Sim0
$\bar{\sigma}_b$	10.7	17.0	35.4	27.1
$r_{\Delta,1}$	-18.7±9.4	-10.1±9.3	-1.4±11.1	-3.5±9.7
s_Δ	20.9	13.8	11.1	10.4
$r_{\Delta,2}$	-13.0±10.0	-5.8±9.8	0.4±11.3	-1.2±10.0
s_Δ	16.5	11.4	11.3	10.1
$r_{\Delta,3}$	-11.8±8.4	-4.4±7.7	1.9±9.8	0.3±8.2
s_Δ	14.5	8.9	10.0	8.2
$r_{\Delta,4}$	-1.8±4.0	-0.4±3.5	0.6±2.8	0.3±2.8
s_Δ	4.4	3.5	2.8	2.8
Head	Sim10	Sim30	Sim50	Sim0
$\bar{\sigma}_b$	16.1	26.1	62.0	58.3
$r_{\Delta,1}$	-29.2±3.7	-19.9±6.9	4.9±13.8	20.9±11.1
s_Δ	29.5	21.0	14.6	23.7
$r_{\Delta,2}$	-27.8±3.8	-18.8±7.0	4.8±13.8	19.4±11.0
s_Δ	28.0	20.0	14.6	22.3
$r_{\Delta,3}$	-23.7±3.3	-14.4±4.3	10.2±9.2	25.7±6.0
s_Δ	23.9	15.0	13.7	26.4
$r_{\Delta,4}$	-6.3±2.1	-4.7±1.7	0.2±2.0	3.0±2.4
s_Δ	6.7	5.0	2.0	3.9

Tab. 7.1 summarizes the results of the systematic error evaluation achieved for the three phantoms. The average pixel noise values $\bar{\sigma}_b$ in HU are listed for the different phantoms and reconstruction kernels. This average pixel noise was determined by averaging over the standard deviation image achieved from the Monte-Carlo simulation. In addition, the relative systematic errors are listed for four different cases:

1. All covariances are neglected, giving $r_{\Delta,1}$ and $s_{\Delta,1}$.

2. The covariances during backprojection are neglected, giving $r_{\Delta,2}$ and $s_{\Delta,2}$.

3. The covariances between neighboring projections during backprojection are neglected, giving $r_{\Delta,3}$ and $s_{\Delta,3}$.

4. All covariances proposed in the method presented here are taken into account, giving $r_{\Delta,4}$ and $s_{\Delta,4}$.

The relative systematic errors are averaged over the whole image domain and quoted in percent, together with their standard deviations. Additionally, the L2-norm errors are quoted as well.

For better judging the results the standard deviation images obtained from the analytic noise propagation and from the Monte-Carlo can be compared in Fig. 7.5. Additionally, horizontal and vertical lineplots through the center of the standard deviation images are displayed in Fig. 7.7, Fig. 7.8, and Fig. 7.9. The accuracy of the four different configurations of the algorithm can here be compared visually for the different phantoms and reconstruction kernels.

It is evident, that good results over the full range of convolution kernels can only be achieved by considering the covariances during the convolution and backprojection processes. This can be seen from the quantitative evaluation as well as from the lineplots through the standard deviation images. Without considering the correlations introduced to the data during the processing, the noise is under- or overestimated, sometimes up to more than 40%. This estimation error cannot be adjusted by a correction factor or shift, because the deviation of the errors within the image strongly varies. The consideration of the correlations introduced during rebinning for the convolution process only leads to improvements for smoother reconstruction kernels. It can be clearly seen from the lineplots, that especially for Sim50 and Sim0 nearly no changes are noticable (regarding the magenta and cyan curves). The reason is that the smoother kernels have a wider spatial extension and, therefore, the correlations within the neighborhoods have more influence. Taking into account the correlation between neighboring channels during the interpolation performed within the backprojections improves the noise estimation in all cases (regarding the red curve in the lineplots). The additional consideration of correlations between neighboring projections, when summing up the contributions from all directions to the local noise variance in the backprojection, has again a larger impact if smoother reconstruction kernels are used. Another observation is that the influence is higher the farther the distance of the pixel to the iso-center. This can be understood regarding the ACCFs of the smooth Sim10 and sharp Sim0 kernel plotted in Fig. 7.4. The larger the distance of the currently reconstructed pixel to the iso-center, the larger is the distance between the channels of two neighboring projections contributing to that pixel. While the ACCF is still not 0 for a smooth kernel, there is no noticeable correlation between these samples in case of a sharp kernel. If all the correlations are taken into account for the noise propagation the method shows good accuracy with an average relative error below 6.3% for the head phantom and even below 2% for the shoulder phantom. The L2-norm errors are in about the same range between 6.7% for very smooth reconstruction kernels and close to 2% for sharp reconstruction kernels.

7.3.3 Real Data

In addition to the evaluation based on simulated data, some experiments with data acquired at a Siemens Definition CT scanner were performed. For estimating noise in the projections

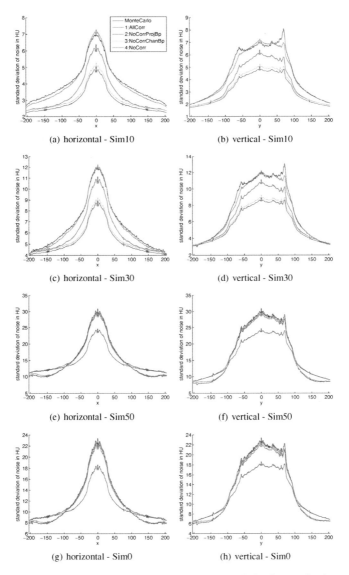

(a) horizontal - Sim10

(b) vertical - Sim10

(c) horizontal - Sim30

(d) vertical - Sim30

(e) horizontal - Sim50

(f) vertical - Sim50

(g) horizontal - Sim0

(h) vertical - Sim0

Figure 7.7: Horizontal and vertical cuts through standard deviation images for thorax phantom - comparison of Monte-Carlo results to four different cases of analytical noise propagation for four different reconstruction kernels.

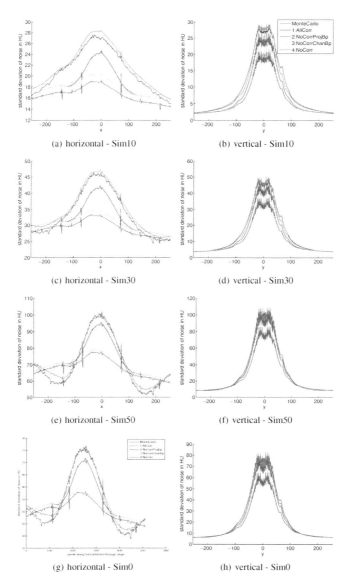

(a) horizontal - Sim10

(b) vertical - Sim10

(c) horizontal - Sim30

(d) vertical - Sim30

(e) horizontal - Sim50

(f) vertical - Sim50

(g) horizontal - Sim0

(h) vertical - Sim0

Figure 7.8: Horizontal and vertical cuts through standard deviation images for shoulder region of thorax phantom - comparison of Monte-Carlo results to four different cases of analytical noise propagation for four different reconstruction kernels.

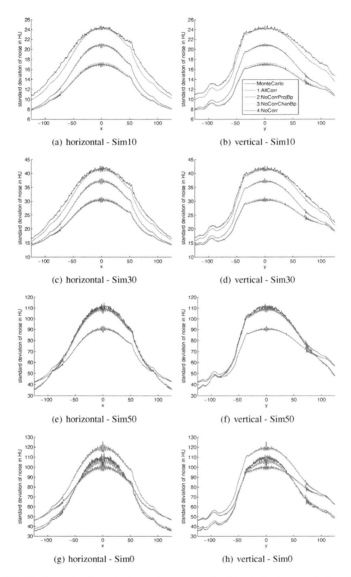

(a) horizontal - Sim10

(b) vertical - Sim10

(c) horizontal - Sim30

(d) vertical - Sim30

(e) horizontal - Sim50

(f) vertical - Sim50

(g) horizontal - Sim0

(h) vertical - Sim0

Figure 7.9: Horizontal and vertical cuts through standard deviation images for head phantom - comparison of Monte-Carlo results to four different cases of analytical noise propagation for four different reconstruction kernels.

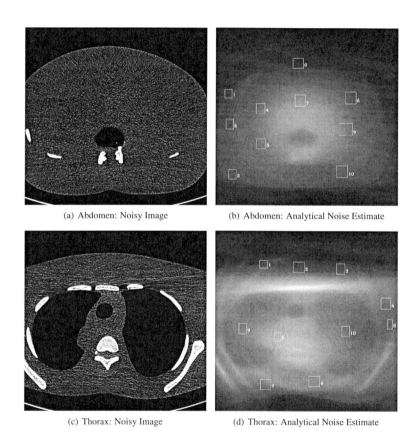

(a) Abdomen: Noisy Image   (b) Abdomen: Analytical Noise Estimate

(c) Thorax: Noisy Image   (d) Thorax: Analytical Noise Estimate

Figure 7.10: Experiments with real data acquired at a Siemens Definition CT scanner (300mm FOV, B40f, display: w=50, c=400), together with analytical noise estimates (display: w=50, c=80). The pixel regions used for evaluation of local standard deviations in noisy image and average standard deviation from analytic noise propagation are shown with their respective numbers.

of scanned CT data, a physical noise model for the projection data needs to be calibrated in advance. As already mentioned in Section 2.4.1, the system specific parameters c and σ_e^2 can be determined by measuring noise and signal strength at various fluxes. Especially, if the CT scanner is equipped with a bowtie-filter, each detector channel has an individual set of parameters. Eccentric positioned water cylinders of different diameters were used for the calibration measurements performed at 120 kV and 300 mA. At the same scanner two different anatomical phantoms were scanned again at 120 kV and 300 mA. The images reconstructed at a FOV of 25 cm with a medium sharp body kernel (B40f) are shown in Fig. 7.10. The standard deviation of noise was measured in 10 different homogeneous image regions and was compared to the average standard deviation of noise from the analytical noise propagation, averaged over the same pixel region.

Table 7.2: Comparison of standard deviation of noise evaluated in homogeneous image regions of reconstructed noisy CT image ref and mean standard deviation in this pixel region of the analytic noise propagation $\bar{\sigma}_{rec}$. The standard deviations are given in HU, the relative error r_Δ is given in percent.

Abdomen	1	2	3	4	5	6	7	8	9	10
$\bar{\sigma}_{ref}$	34.8	38.4	36.1	44.5	52.2	32.9	57.8	40.9	50.8	45.6
$\bar{\sigma}_{rec}$	34.5	38.6	36.3	46.2	47.0	33.1	54.0	42.4	49.9	41.7
$r_{\Delta,r}$	-1.0	0.5	-1.1	3.9	-10	0.5	-6.5	3.8	-1.8	-8.5

Thorax	1	2	3	4	5	6	7	8	9	10
$\bar{\sigma}_{ref}$	39.1	41.4	42.7	46.5	43.9	55.3	47.3	67.7	50.5	47.9
$\bar{\sigma}_{rec}$	37.6	38.4	39.3	45.1	42.5	50.6	46.0	59.7	47.8	47.1
$r_{\Delta,r}$	-3.9	-7.2	-8.1	-2.9	-3.3	-8.4	-2.7	-11.8	-5.4	-1.7

The standard deviation of noise evaluated in local neighborhoods of about 600 pixels is here denoted as $\bar{\sigma}_{ref}$. These reference noise values are compared to the standard deviation of noise from the analytic noise propagation, respectively averaged over the different local neighborhoods, and is denoted as $\bar{\sigma}_{rec}$. The maximum standard deviation of the computed standard deviation values within the small pixel regions was in all cases below 2 HU in case of the abdomen image and below 1 HU for the thorax image. A comparison of the standard deviations is presented in Tab. 7.2. In addition to the standard deviations the relative deviation of the reference noise and the computed standard deviations is computed for the different image regions:

$$r_{\Delta,r} = \frac{\bar{\sigma}_{rec} - \bar{\sigma}_{ref}}{\bar{\sigma}_{ref}}. \tag{7.46}$$

It can be seen that the noise estimate from the analytic noise propagation fits well to the standard deviation evaluated in homogeneous image regions. The average relative deviation is about -2.3% in case of the abdomen image and -5.5% in case of the thorax image. The maximum relative deviation was about -12%. In most of the cases the local standard deviation of noise is slightly underestimated.

7.4 Conclusions

In this chapter, a fast method for noise-propagation through indirect fan-beam FBP reconstruction with rebinning to parallel-beam geometry was proposed. Due to the fact that the rebinning step and all further processing steps correlate the input data, approximative models based on linear shift-invariant systems were developed for estimating the covariance terms needed for the variance computations. The proposed methodology has been validated by Monte-Carlo and demonstrates good accuracy with an average relative error below 6.6%. It was observed that with increasing sharpness of the used reconstruction kernels a lower systematic error of about 2% can be obtained. The main limiting factor is seen in the approximation in the covariance terms. The better spatially concentrated the involved operations work, the better the wide-sense-stationarity assumptions for the ACCF computation holds, which explains the better results for sharper kernels. Due to the fact that the ultimate goal is to compute a standard-deviation image for post-processing purposes, the method was additionally tested with respect to statistical errors. Even if the noise variance in the fan-beam projections was estimated from noisy projections of a single noise realization, only negligible differences below 0.1% were observed, compared to the case of perfectly known variance in the projections. Experiments with real accquired CT data showed that in combination with a calibrated physical noise model the proposed analytic noise propagation can be used for estimating the local standard deviation in the reconstructed image. The relative deviation between the computed local standard deviation of noise and the standard deviation of noise evaluated in small homogeneous image regions is below 12% for all image regions evaluated for both real scans under investigation. Furthermore, the introduced approximations allow a fast and easy implementation. Especially for the focus of application, the adaptation of post-processing methods to the special noise, properties in CT, the presented noise propagation method is precise enough and shows stable results also for estimated variances in the projections from a single noisy measurement. The computational performance of the noise propagation is comparable to another reconstruction.

Of course, some simplifying approximations for the noise model in the fan-beam projections were used for the simulations and in the physical noise model. First of all, monochromatic X-ray beams were assumed, which is unrealistic for practical systems. It is, however, very common to approximate the polyenergetic X-rays measured at the detector by only considering an effective energy and an average number of photons, which is again very close to the simple model used here. Furthermore, electronics noise was neglected for the simulations. In real systems, electronics noise is usually very small compared to quantum noise, if the X-ray flux is high enough. Consequently, only for very low doses electronics noise plays a role. In the physical noise model that was used for the real data electronics noise was considered. Obviously electronics noise, which is usually modeled as a Gaussian noise floor does not severely influence the accuracy of the presented method. Further, noise in the fan-beam projections was considered to be perfectly uncorrelated. This assumption only holds as long as tube-current variations, cross-talk at the detector and afterglow are negligibly small. In real systems the noise in the measured projections is usually very small, but there are small correlations between neighboring channels and projections. Although, these correlations were neglected in case of the real scans, the noise estimates are still reliable enough for the desired post-processing application. For future investigations, it is also possible to include the correlation of the input data into the proposed methodology. As long as these correlations can be modeled by a linear shift-invariant system, the proposed methodology can still be applied with only little changes. The ACCF of the fan-beam projections is then no longer a delta function, which is used for the covariance computation during the rebinning and thus the covariances no longer cancel out in the first processing step. Consequently, the ACCF needs to be updated after the intermediate rebinning steps, too.

Chapter 8

Orientation Dependent Noise Propagation for Adaptive Anisotropic Filtering

As already indicated in the last chapter, precise knowledge of the local noise variance would help in adapting various post-processing methods to the non-stationary noise in CT. Noise reduction methods can for example make use of this additional knowledge and adapt to the local contrast-to-noise ratio. Ideally, post-processing methods should also account for the local correlation of noise. Improved noise suppression can be obtained knowing the correlation of noise within the local neighborhoods that are used for filtering. Averaging uncorrelated values leads to a stronger noise suppression than averaging values that are strongly correlated. The computation of image covariances has been investigated for direct fan-beam reconstruction in [Wund 08]. It is also possible to approximate the covariances in images reconstructed with indirect fan-beam FBP using the approximation presented in Chapter 7.2.5. Nevertheless, such computations are very time consuming if they are performed pixel-wise for the whole image domain and, thus, not useful for image denoising purposes in practice. Therefore, this chapter presents an extension of the analytic noise propagation presented in the last chapter that additionally gives some information about the correlation of noise without computing covariances. Additionally, the adaptation of a bilateral filter to the non-stationary, correlated noise is investigated.

In a preliminary approach [Bors 08b], the local noise variance was split up into its horizontal and vertical contributions. The estimated noise variances in the projections are weighted with sine-/cosine-squares of the respective parallel projection angles and separately propagated through the indirect fan-beam reconstruction, as described in Chapter 7. The overall local noise variance is the sum of horizontal and vertical variance contributions. The ratio between horizontal and vertical contribution to the local variance is then used for adapting the bilateral filter. The Gaussian range filter can, e. g., be stretched or suppressed along the x/y-direction. The remaining problem is that diagonally directed noise grains evenly split up into its horizontal and vertical contributions according to this orientation separation based on just the horizontal and vertical directions. As a result the filter in these special cases remains an isotropic filter and the desired effect gets lost.

The idea of the improved approach, presented here, is: Per pixel the direction is determined that mostly contributes to the local noise variance. This is the direction for which the X-ray had to travel through most or densest material. It will be shown that this is at the same time closely related to the direction of highest correlation within a local neighborhood. Instead of determining just the horizontal and vertical contribution to the overall local noise variance, the contribution in direction of the highest correlation and orthogonal to it is computed. This means that for each pixel a specific separation into two directions is performed. Based on these noise contributions and the corresponding angle pointing out the orientation of the noise grain at a certain position, a noise adaptive filtering can be performed that takes into account the noise correlations. The filter is adapted such that strongest filtering is applied orthogonal to the direction of highest correlation. The concept of bilateral filtering, a simple and widely used technique, is used here as a basis for noise adaptive edge-preserving filtering.

8.1 Methodology Overview

The flowchart of the methodology is presented in Fig. 8.1 including intermediate results for an example slice of a real scan. The method splits up into the following parts:

1. The CT image is reconstructed using indirect fan-beam FBP reconstruction.

2. The noise variance in the fan-beam projections is estimated according to a calibrated physical noise model, as described in Section 2.4.1.

3. The local noise variance is computed based on the analytic noise propagation for indirect fan-beam FBP, as described in Chapter 7. At the same time the direction of strongest correlation is determined for each image pixel.

4. Based on the computed direction of strongest correlation a pixelwise separation of the overall noise variance into the direction of strongest correlation and orthogonal to that is computed. The separation is obtained by a modified noise propagation method where sine-/cosine-square weights are used during the backprojection of the variances.

5. The orientation dependent noise estimates in the image domain and the image pointing out the direction of highest correlation are used for post-processing of the reconstructed CT image. Here, a noise adaptive bilateral filtering is proposed as an example application.

In the following the determination of the direction of strongest correlation and the locally dependent separation of the noise variance to the contribution along the direction of highest correlation and orthogonal to it are described more in detail. After that the adaptation of the bilateral filter to the non-stationary and non-isotropic noise in the CT image will show how this additional information can be used for improving the signal-to-noise ratio in the image.

8.2 Orientation Dependent Noise Propagation

In Chapter 7 an algorithm for the computation of local noise variances has been provided. Given the noisy projection values, a simple (calibrated) noise model can be used for esti-

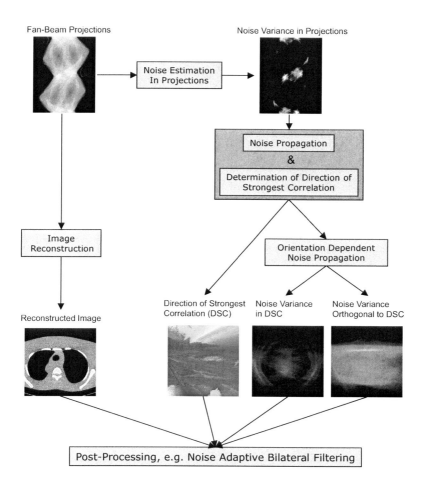

Figure 8.1: Methodology overview.

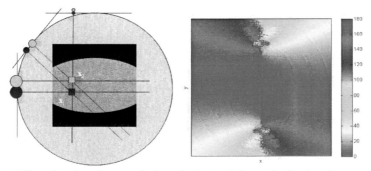

(a) Illustration of covariance contributions. (b) Angle pointing out the direction of strongest correlation.

Figure 8.2: Illustration of covariance computation and determination of direction of strongest correlation.

mating noise in the projections. Starting from this, the noise variance can be propagated through the complete reconstruction pipeline.

In addition to the local variance, the correlation of noise is now analyzed. The computation of covariances is possible, as explained in Section 7.2.5. However, this computation is rather time consuming. In this section, another possibility for getting information about the noise correlation, without computation of covariances will be described. In a first step, it will be shown that for each pixel in the image the direction of strongest correlation can be easily determined. With this direction the first principal axis of the local noise grain is obtained.

The second part of this section then describes a method for separating the local variance into two noise contributions. This separation can be performed uniformly for the whole image, e. g., into a horizontal and vertical contribution. As already mentioned above, this has the drawback that in some cases no information about the noise anisotropy can be gained. Therefore, an extended approach where a pixel specific separation into the direction of strongest correlation and orthogonal to that is computed is introduced.

8.2.1 Direction of Strongest Correlation

The non-isotropic noise property in reconstructed CT images can be mainly derived from the non-stationary noise in the projections. As explained in chapter Chapter 7, the variances in the projections are backprojected for computing the local noise variances in the reconstructed images, according to Eq. (7.26), which can also be written as:

$$\text{Var}(\mu(\mathbf{x})) = \Delta\theta^2 \sum_{i=1}^{N_{\pi p}} v(\theta_i, \mathbf{x}). \tag{8.1}$$

For each pixel position $\mathbf{x}$, the variance contributions

$$v(\theta_i, \mathbf{x}) = \text{Var}(P_i^{\text{fil}}(\mathbf{x})) + \sum_{i=1}^{N_{\pi p}} \sum_{j=1}^{j_{max}} \left(\text{Cov}(P_i^{\text{fil}}(\mathbf{x}), P_{i+j}^{\text{fil}}(\mathbf{x})) + \text{Cov}(P_i^{\text{fil}}(\mathbf{x}), P_{i-j}^{\text{fil}}(\mathbf{x})) \right). \quad (8.2)$$

coming from the parallel-beam projections at different projection angles θ_i are collected, or summed up, as illustrated in Fig. 8.2(a). The variance $\text{Var}(P_i^{\text{fil}}(\mathbf{x}))$ and covariances $\text{Cov}(P_i^{\text{fil}}(\mathbf{x}), P_j^{\text{fil}}(\mathbf{x}))$ in Eq. (8.2) are computed according to Eq. (7.30) and Eq. (7.28). Because of this backprojection process, all image pixels that are placed along the backprojection line $L(\theta, t)$ receive the same contribution from the projection at angle θ. The correlations between neighboring projections (in direction of θ) and within a projection (in direction of t) are rather small. Examples of estimated auto correlation coefficient functions of noise in the projections after rebinning and convolution were shown in the previous chapter in Fig. 7.4. Because of the small spatial extension of the ACCF most of the contributing variances to the overall variance at a pixel positioned at $\mathbf{x}_1$ and another pixel at $\mathbf{x}_2$ are uncorrelated, except for the variance backprojected along the straight line defined by $\mathbf{x}_1$ and $\mathbf{x}_2$. The correlation between the two pixels is stronger the higher the backprojected variance along this straight line is. If different pixels with the same distance to the reference pixel are considered, it becomes clear that the direction of strongest correlation is given by the direction from which the strongest contribution to the overall variance is collected during backprojection of the projection variances. This means that during the computation of the local noise variance, the projection angle with the strongest contribution to the noise variance of the actual pixel can be determined:

$$\theta_{max}(\mathbf{x}) = \text{argmax}_{\theta_i} \left\{ v(\theta_i, \mathbf{x}) \right\}. \quad (8.3)$$

From the determined angle $\theta_{max}(\mathbf{x})$ in the range of $[0, \pi]$ the direction vector

$$\breve{\theta}_{max}(\mathbf{x}) = (\cos(\theta_{max}(\mathbf{x})), \sin(\theta_{max}(\mathbf{x})))^T \quad (8.4)$$

points in the direction of strongest correlation. It points out the first principal axis of the noise grain, meaning the direction in which the noise grain has its largest spatial extension. In case of an isotropic noise grain $\breve{\theta}_{max}(\mathbf{x})$ can be an arbitrary direction. An example for the pixel-wise determined direction of strongest correlation is displayed in Fig. 8.2(b) for the ellipse shown in Fig. 8.2(a). The angle $\theta_{max}(\mathbf{x})$ is displayed color-coded.

8.2.2 Orthogonal Separation of Noise Variance

With the above presented analysis, the direction of strongest correlation can be computed from the noise estimates in the projections. There is, however, no information given, if the noise grain is really anisotropic or if the contributions from all directions are the same. In order to obtain information about the noise anisotropy, a pixelwise separation of the noise variance into its contributions from two orthogonal directions is computed.

The idea of the presented approach is based on the observation that the noise variance in the parallel projection at angle θ mainly contributes to the noise variance in the image orthogonal to the backprojection direction. This means that if the projection at angle θ is very noisy and is backprojected, any line orthogonal to the backprojection line is very

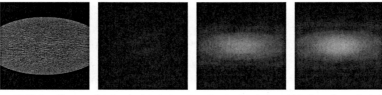

(a) Noisy ellipse | (b) Standard deviation of noise in horizontal direction. | (c) Standard deviation of noise in vertical direction. | (d) Overall standard diviation of noise.

Figure 8.3: Example of horizontal and vertical noise contributions for elliptical water phantom.

noisy, too. Any line that is parallel to the backprojection line, on the other hand, is inferred by the same error from the current projection and thus shows a constant error along this line with respect to this projection direction. The theoretical basis for this observation builds the Fourier-Slice-Theorem, as described in Section 2.2. If only one parallel-beam projection is considered the one-dimensional Fourier transformation of the projection at angle θ is equivalent to the two-dimensional Fourier transformation of the reconstructed function along the line through the origin in direction of $\gamma = \theta - \pi/2$. As discussed before, the noise in CT can be assumed to be additive and zero-mean. Because of the linearity of the FBP, noise can be considered separately. If the parallel-beam projection acquired at angle θ just consists of noise, the reconstruction shows noise in the orthogonal direction of $\gamma = \theta - \pi/2$, because the two-dimensional Fourier Transformation of the reconstruction is only non-zero along this one line. This observation is useful for separating the overall noise variance into its contributions to certain directions, e. g. the horizontal and vertical directions [Bors 08b]. As described above, the projections with θ close to 0 mainly contribute to the noise in vertical direction in the image (y-direction) and projections with θ close to $\pi/2$ to noise in horizontal direction (x-direction). By weighting the variance in the projections with sine- and cosine-squares of the parallel projection angle, the overall noise variance can be split up into two parts:

$$
\begin{aligned}
\mathrm{Var}(\mu(\mathbf{x})) &= \Delta\theta^2 \sum_{i=1}^{N_{\pi p}} v(\theta_i, \mathbf{x}) = \Delta\theta^2 \sum_{i=1}^{N_{\pi p}} (\sin^2\theta_i + \cos^2\theta_i)\, v(\theta_i, \mathbf{x}) = \\
&= \underbrace{\Delta\theta^2 \sum_{i=1}^{N_{\pi p}} \sin^2\theta_i\, v(\theta_i, \mathbf{x})}_{\mathrm{Var_H}(\mu(\mathbf{x}))} + \underbrace{\Delta\theta^2 \sum_{i=1}^{N_{\pi p}} \cos^2\theta_i\, v(\theta_i, \mathbf{x})}_{\mathrm{Var_V}(\mu(\mathbf{x}))} .
\end{aligned}
\tag{8.5}
$$

The variance contribution $\mathrm{Var_H}(\mu(\mathbf{x}))$ to the horizontal direction is computed by applying sine-square weights depending on the parallel projection angle during the backprojection process. Accordingly, the vertical variance contribution $\mathrm{Var_V}(\mu(\mathbf{x}))$ is obtained by using cosine-square weights for the backprojection. Based on the horizontal and vertical variances for the reconstructed attenuation values, orientation dependent variance images of the reconstructed Hounsfield values can be computed, based on Eq. (7.32) and Eq. (7.33):

$$\sigma_{\mathrm{H}}^2(\mathbf{x}) = \mathrm{Var}_{\mathrm{H}}(\mu(\mathbf{x})) \left(\frac{1000}{\mu_w} \ \mathrm{HU} \right)^2, \tag{8.6}$$

and

$$\sigma_{\mathrm{V}}^2(\mathbf{x}) = \mathrm{Var}_{\mathrm{V}}(\mu(\mathbf{x})) \left(\frac{1000}{\mu_w} \ \mathrm{HU} \right)^2, \tag{8.7}$$

Clearly, these noise estimates depend on the local position $\mathbf{x}$. A noise estimation vector:

$$\hat{\sigma}(\mathbf{x}) = (\sigma_{\mathrm{H}}(\mathbf{x}), \sigma_{\mathrm{V}}(\mathbf{x}))^T \tag{8.8}$$

is now given for every pixel position $\mathbf{x}$. By construction, the noise variance in the reconstructed CT image can be expressed as:

$$\sigma^2(\mathbf{x}) = \sigma_{\mathrm{H}}^2(\mathbf{x}) + \sigma_{\mathrm{V}}^2(\mathbf{x}). \tag{8.9}$$

This means that at position $\mathbf{x}$ the standard deviation of noise $\sigma(\mathbf{x})$ is given by the norm of the noise vector defined in Eq. (8.8). An example for such a separation into horizontal and vertical noise contribution is shown in Fig. 8.3. It can be seen clearly that noise in horizontal direction is much lower than noise in vertical direction for the elliptical water phantom.

The above presented theory allows the separation of the noise variance into two orthogonal directions. The drawback, however, is that noise sometimes equally contributes to both directions, e.g. in case of perfectly diagonally directed noise grains. Thus, no information about the anisotropy of noise can be gained anymore. Therefore, an extended method for noise separation is described here. The local noise variance is split up into its contribution in direction of strongest noise correlation at the local position and orthogonal to that. Hence, the separation is done specifically for each single pixel position. The idea of the extended method is as following: In a first step the overall local noise variance $\sigma^2(\mathbf{x})$ is computed as described in Chapter 7. The direction of strongest correlation $\theta_{\max}(\mathbf{x})$ can be determined simultaneously to the computation of the overall local noise variance $\sigma^2(\mathbf{x})$, as described in Section 8.2.1. Then a pixelwise separation of the local variance into the contribution orthogonal and along the direction of strongest correlation is computed.

The variance contribution orthogonal to the direction of strongest correlation is obtained using pixelwise backprojection weights depending on the sum of the parallel projection angle θ and the angle pointing out the direction of strongest correlation $\theta_{max}(\mathbf{x})$ at position $\mathbf{x}$:

$$\sigma_{\perp}^2(\mathbf{x}) = \left(\Delta\theta \frac{1000}{\mu_w} \ \mathrm{HU} \right)^2 \sum_{i=1}^{N_{\pi p}} \cos^2(\theta_i + \theta_{max}(\mathbf{x}))\, v(\theta_i, \mathbf{x}). \tag{8.10}$$

Analogously, the variance contribution in direction of strongest correlation is given by:

$$\sigma_{\|}^2(\mathbf{x}) = \left(\Delta\theta \frac{1000}{\mu_w} \ \mathrm{HU} \right)^2 \sum_{i=1}^{N_{\pi p}} \sin^2(\theta_i + \theta_{max}(\mathbf{x}))\, v(\theta_i, \mathbf{x}). \tag{8.11}$$

The overall noise variance can again be expressed as pointwise sum of the two noise contributions:

$$\sigma^2(\mathbf{x}) = \sigma_\perp^2(\mathbf{x}) + \sigma_\parallel^2(\mathbf{x}). \tag{8.12}$$

If the overall noise variance has already been computed, only one additional weighted backprojection of the variances is necessary for getting the noise separation.

8.3   Noise Adaptive Bilateral Filtering

For the adaptation of anisotropic edge-preserving filtering methods to the noise characteristics in CT, two things are of main interest. The local noise variance should be considered, because noise in CT is non-stationary. Secondly, the local noise correlation should be taken into account, because noise is non-isotropic. Here, a noise adaptive method that is mainly based on the idea of bilateral filtering [Toma 98], a simple and widely used edge-preserving noise reduction approach, will be discussed.

In case of bilateral filtering, the image $f(\mathbf{x})$ is smoothed by non-linear averaging in local neighborhoods. During averaging, in addition to the geometric closeness of image pixels, also the photometric similarity between the pixel values is taken into consideration. The filtered image $\tilde{f}(\mathbf{x})$ is computed as follows:

$$\tilde{f}(\mathbf{x}) = \frac{1}{n(\mathbf{x})} \sum_{\mathbf{x'}} f(\mathbf{x'}) c(\mathbf{x}, \mathbf{x'}) s(f(\mathbf{x}), f(\mathbf{x'})), \tag{8.13}$$

where $n(\mathbf{x})$ is needed for normalization and is given by:

$$n(\mathbf{x}) = \sum_{\mathbf{x}} c(\mathbf{x}, \mathbf{x'}) s(f(\mathbf{x}), f(\mathbf{x'})). \tag{8.14}$$

The function $c(\mathbf{x}, \mathbf{x'})$, also called domain filter, takes into account the geometric closeness of the actual pixel at position $\mathbf{x}$ and a neighboring pixel $\mathbf{x'}$. The function $s(f(\mathbf{x}), f(\mathbf{x'}))$, in the following called range filter, brings in the edge-preserving characteristic of the filter. It takes into account the photometric closeness of the image pixels during averaging. In the standard approach both, the range and domain filter, are usually chosen as simple Gaussian filters [Toma 98]. The domain filter decreases with increasing Euclidean distance between the neighboring pixels and the range filter decreases with increasing difference between the pixel values. The standard deviations of these filters are the steerable parameters that control the amount of noise reduction on the one hand, but also the edge-preservation capability on the other hand. The direct application of the standard bilateral filter to reconstructed CT images shows unconvincing results in most cases. Due to the non-stationarity of noise, the selection of a global parameter for the range filter is problematic. The noise amplitude varies in different image regions, and, thus, image regions with lower noise level might be smoothed well, while noise is visibly remaining in other regions. The range filter should be adapted to the local contrast-to-noise level. Further, in case of strongly anisotropic noise grains, the filter should try to stretch and rotate, such that a higher number of uncorrelated values are used for averaging.

8.3.1 Domain Filtering

Taking the anisotropy of noise in reconstructed CT images into consideration, the domain filter is chosen as a multivariate Gaussian filter. It adjusts to the orientation of maximal correlation at the local position and takes into account the local orientation dependent noise variances $\sigma_\perp^2(\mathbf{x})$ and $\sigma_\parallel^2(\mathbf{x})$. The filter is stretch and compressed such that strongest filtering is performed orthogonal to the direction of strongest correlation. The noise adaptive domain filter is defined as:

$$c(\mathbf{x}, \mathbf{x}') = e^{-\frac{1}{2}(\mathbf{x}-\mathbf{x}')^T \Sigma_{\mathbf{x}}^{-1}(\mathbf{x}-\mathbf{x}')}. \tag{8.15}$$

The covariance matrix $\Sigma_{\mathbf{x}}$ controls the degree of anisotropy and the orientation of the filter. It can be written as

$$\Sigma_{\mathbf{x}} = \mathbf{R}_x^T \mathbf{D}_x \mathbf{R}_x, \tag{8.16}$$

where $\mathbf{R}_x$ is a rotation matrix:

$$\mathbf{R}_x = \begin{pmatrix} \cos(\gamma_{\max}(\mathbf{x})) & \sin(\gamma_{\max}(\mathbf{x})) \\ -\sin(\gamma_{\max}(\mathbf{x})) & \cos(\gamma_{\max}(\mathbf{x})) \end{pmatrix} \tag{8.17}$$

and $\mathbf{D}_x$ is a diagonal matrix:

$$\mathbf{D}_x = \begin{pmatrix} \nu_1(\mathbf{x}) & 0 \\ 0 & \nu_2(\mathbf{x}) \end{pmatrix}. \tag{8.18}$$

The decomposition in Eq. (8.16) is the singular value decomposition of the covariance matrix $\Sigma_{\mathbf{x}}$. The principal axes are given by the row-vectors of $\mathbf{R}_x$. Here it can be seen that the first principal axis is rotated such that it points orthogonal to the direction of strongest correlation. The extension of the filter in direction of strongest correlation and orthogonal to it is steered by the singular values in the diagonal matrix $\mathbf{D}_x$. The singular value $\nu_1(\mathbf{x})$ controls the spatial extension of the filter orthogonal to the direction of strongest correlation and $\nu_2(\mathbf{x})$ in direction of strongest correlation. These two values should be chosen based on the orientation dependent variance contributions $\sigma_\perp^2(\mathbf{x})$ and $\sigma_\parallel^2(\mathbf{x})$. If both parts are equivalent an isotropic Gaussian filter is desired. The stronger the two components differ from each other the stronger the filter should be stretched in direction orthogonal to the direction of strongest correlation. We define the singular values based on the ratio of the orientation dependent local variances and the overall local variance:

$$\nu_1(\mathbf{x}) = q^{\left(2\frac{\sigma_\perp^2(\mathbf{x})}{\sigma^2(\mathbf{x})}-1\right)} d^2, \tag{8.19}$$

and

$$\nu_2(\mathbf{x}) = q^{\left(2\frac{\sigma_\parallel^2(\mathbf{x})}{\sigma^2(\mathbf{x})}-1\right)} d^2, \tag{8.20}$$

with parameters $q \in \mathbb{N}$ and $d \in \mathbb{R}$. If the two variances $\sigma_\perp^2(\mathbf{x})$ and $\sigma_\parallel^2(\mathbf{x})$ are equivalent, an isotropic Gaussian filter with standard deviation d is obtained. Otherwise, the parameter q controls the degree of maximum anisotropy of the filter. The spatial extension of the filter orthogonal to the direction of strongest correlation is maximally factor q times higher than along the direction of highest correlation. The above definition of $\nu_1(\mathbf{x})$ and $\nu_2(\mathbf{x})$ ensures that the area under the filter is constant:

$$\int\int e^{-\frac{1}{2}(\mathbf{x}-\mathbf{x}')^T \Sigma_{\mathbf{x}}^{-1}(\mathbf{x}-\mathbf{x}')} dx\, dy \overset{!}{=} \text{const}, \tag{8.21}$$

because the determinant of the matrix $\Sigma_{\mathbf{x}}^{-1}$ is constant, independently from the distribution of the overall variance to the contributions into the two orthogonal directions. The determinant is computed as:

$$\det\left(\Sigma_{\mathbf{x}}^{-1}\right) = \det\left(\Sigma_{\mathbf{x}}\right)^{-1} = \frac{1}{\nu_1(\mathbf{x})\nu_2(\mathbf{x})} = \frac{1}{d^4} \tag{8.22}$$

and consequently ensures the requirement.

8.3.2   Range Filtering

The second part of the bilateral filter is the range filter, which is the edge-preserving component. It takes into account the photometric similarity of neighboring pixels. The larger the difference between the pixel values compared to the noise level, the lower is the impact to the averaging result. With the knowledge of the local variances, the difference between pixel values can be set into relation to the respective standard deviation of the two pixel values. The variance of the difference of the two pixel values can be computed as:

$$\text{Var}(f(\mathbf{x}) - f(\mathbf{x}')) = \sigma^2(\mathbf{x}) + \sigma^2(\mathbf{x}') + 2\text{Cov}(f(\mathbf{x}), f(\mathbf{x}')). \tag{8.23}$$

However, the covariance between the pixels is not known here. As described above, the computation of the covariance matrix is avoided because of computational performance reasons. The correlation of noise has already been incorporated in the design of the domain filter. Therefore, the covariance in Eq. (8.23) is neglected. The range filter is then defined as a Gaussian filter that decreases with increasing local contrast-to-noise ratio:

$$s(f(\mathbf{x}), f(\mathbf{x}')) = e^{-\frac{1}{2}\frac{(f(\mathbf{x})-f(\mathbf{x}'))^2}{(\sigma^2(\mathbf{x})+\sigma^2(\mathbf{x}'))r^2}}. \tag{8.24}$$

The parameter $r \in \mathbb{R}, r > 0$ is used for controlling the amount of noise suppression. With increasing r the range filter allows to take pixels with a larger intensity difference to the reference pixels more into account during averaging. A larger r thus leads to stronger smoothing, but also to lower edge-preservation.

8.4   Experimental Evaluation

For the evaluation of the presented noise reduction method, experiments on simulated and measured data were performed. In this section the proposed noise adaptive filtering method (NABF) is compared to the standard bilateral filtering (SBF) approach with respect to noise and resolution. In a second part of the evaluation section, example images from simulated and measured data are presented.

8.4.1 Noise and Resolution

For the experiments we used the same simulated data and evaluation strategy as already described in Section 6.4.1. In order to achieve smooth MTF curves, several noisy realizations are averaged and the MTF is computed in the averaged image. Preliminary experiments showed, that a contrast-to-noise ratio of about 100 HU is necessary for getting reliable MTF measurements for the phantom used here. Based on that observation the number of images N_c that need to be averaged for the different contrast-to-noise levels can be computed:

$$N_c = \left\lceil \left(\frac{100 \cdot \sigma_c}{c} \right)^2 \right\rceil , \tag{8.25}$$

where σ_c is the standard deviation of noise and c is the contrast of the inlay compared to water, both given in HU. Because of the fact that the noise in the image also changes if the contrast of the inlay strongly varies, the standard deviation of noise σ_c was evaluated in one noisy realization within an ROI inside the cylinder with contrast c for determining the number of images based on Eq. (8.25).

The noise reduction method under investigation was then applied to all the N_c images at a certain contrast c. The MTF was evaluated on the average of all filtered images of the same contrast. From the MTF measured on the edge of the circle a corresponding linear shift-invariant filter can be computed that leads to the same average smoothing in the image as the adaptive filter achieved in average on the edge of the circular inlay, according to Eq. (6.7). Then the standard deviation of noise after adaptive filtering in comparison to standard deviation of noise after application of the linear filter that leads to the same average resolution at the inlay can be investigated.

The NRR (see Eq. (6.9)) and SNRG (see Eq. (6.10)) are then compared between the SBF and NABF. The SBF simply uses a Gaussian range and domain filter, where the standard deviations for both are the input parameters to the algorithm. These two parameters are constant over the whole image domain. The NABF introduced above turns into a SBF, if the standard deviations for the two orthogonal directions given for every image point are equivalent and constant over the whole image domain. Then the angle pointing out the direction of strongest correlation has no effect to the filtering result, because the same isotropic domain filter is computed for every image pixel. For determining a reasonable parameter for the range filter, the average noise variance $\bar{\sigma}^2_{\text{phan}}$ within the elliptical phantom was computed. The standard deviation images were then defined to be of constant value $\sigma^2_\perp(\mathbf{x}) = \sigma^2_\parallel(\mathbf{x}) = \frac{1}{2}\bar{\sigma}^2_{\text{phan}}$ for the whole image domain. The SBF with parameters ($q = 2$, $d = 3$, $r = 2$) was then compared to two configurations of the proposed noise adaptive bilateral filter ($q = 2$, $d = 3$, $r = 1$ and $r = 2$). Examples of filtered images are shown in Fig. 8.4.

A comparison of the MTFs computed for SBF and NABF is shown in Fig. 8.5. The MTF in the original noise-free image is compared to the MTFs computed from filtered images. Adaptive filters lead to different amounts of smoothing for different contrast-to-noise ratios at the edge of the circular object. Therefore, the MTFs are plotted for the different contrasts (1000, 100, 60 and 20 HU). Additionally, the MTF resulting from the application of an isotropic Gaussian filter with $d = 3$ is shown. This gives the lower limit the MTF may reach if the range filter does not show any effect ($r \to \infty$) and the bilateral filter turns into a simple Gaussian domain filter. For all three cases it can be clearly seen

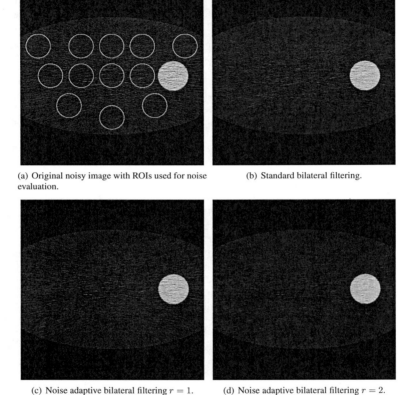

(a) Original noisy image with ROIs used for noise evaluation.

(b) Standard bilateral filtering.

(c) Noise adaptive bilateral filtering $r = 1$.

(d) Noise adaptive bilateral filtering $r = 2$.

Figure 8.4: Elliptical water phantom with circular inlay (here with contrast of 100 HU) used for noise and resolution analysis. The regions used for noise evaluation are marked in the original noisy image (a). The image after application of a standard bilateral filter is shown in (b). Filtering results from two configurations of the proposed noise adaptive filter are shown in (c) and (d).

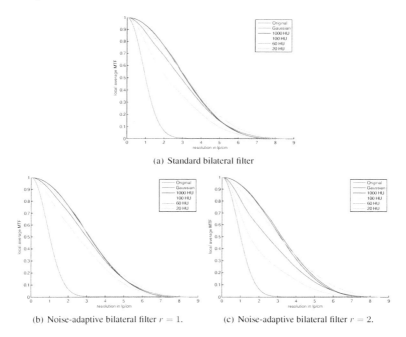

(a) Standard bilateral filter

(b) Noise-adaptive bilateral filter $r = 1$.   (c) Noise-adaptive bilateral filter $r = 2$.

Figure 8.5: Comparison of MTF computed in the averaged filtered images at different contrasts. The standard bilateral filter is compared to two configurations of the proposed method.

that for a very high contrast-to-noise ratio the edge is not smoothed and the MTF is close to the original one. With decreasing contrast, the edges can no longer be perfectly preserved and the edges become smoothed. With increasing parameter r the smoothing at the edge is increased for lower contrast levels. The loss of resolution at the edges in case of the standard bilateral filter, shown in Fig. 8.5(a), is slightly stronger than for the noise adaptive bilateral filter $r = 1$, shown in Fig. 8.5(b). Although the input parameters q, d and r are the same for Fig. 8.5(a), and Fig. 8.5(c). It should, however, be reminded that the nice statistical interpretation of the range filter does not hold for the standard bilateral filter. The local variances are not taken into account and, therefore, the parameter r does not mean that an averaging over pixels that have an intensity difference of more than r times the local standard deviation is avoided. The standard deviation close to the circular object is underestimated by using the constant noise estimate $\bar{\sigma}_{\text{phan}}^2$ for the whole image domain, what means that effectively a much lower filtering effect is obtained close to the edge of the circular inlay with the standard bilateral filter than with the noise adaptive bilateral filter using the same set of parameters q, d and r.

For all the different MTFs presented in Fig. 8.5 the corresponding linear filters that need to be applied to the original image in order to get the same average smoothing at the edge were computed. After the application of the linear filter the noise reduction rate and SNR-gain was compared between the different configurations and the different contrast levels. The results of the noise-resolution analysis are summarized in Tab. 8.1.

Table 8.1: Contrast dependent noise-resolution analysis.

Original Noisy Image	20 HU	60 HU	100 HU	1000 HU
σ_{orig} in HU	17.0±4.0	16.8±3.6	17.1±4.0	20.5±6.4
Standard Bilateral Filter	20 HU	60 HU	100 HU	1000 HU
σ_{fil} in HU	10.8±4.3	10.6±3.8	10.9±4.3	13.3±6.9
NRR in %	38.7±9.6	38.7±10.7	39.2±10.6	40.2±13.1
SNRG in %	7.6±14.7	35.9±11.0	39.0±10.6	40.0±13.1
Noise Adaptive Bilateral Filter ($r = 1$)	20 HU	60 HU	100 HU	1000 HU
σ in HU	12.9±2.9	12.6±2.4	13.0±2.9	15.6±4.6
NRR in %	23.9±1.4	24.5±2.2	24.1±1.8	23.7±2.2
SNRG in %	-0.7±4.0	27.5±5.2	36.4±4.6	24.0±6.1
Noise Adaptive Bilateral Filter ($r = 2$)	20 HU	60 HU	100 HU	1000 HU
σ_{fil} in HU	7.5±1.5	7.3±1.1	7.6±1.6	9.2±2.5
NRR in %	55.0±2.0	54.9±2.1	55.5±2.2	54.8±2.4
SNRG in %	2.4±4.0	46.1±2.8	54.9±2.2	54.8±2.4

From this quantitative analysis, it can be seen that the standard bilateral filter does not take into account the local noise statistics. As can be seen in Fig. 8.4(b), noise in the image is removed quite well in average. There are, however, strong variations between the different regions within the elliptical phantom. At the outer borders noise is strongly removed, while in the center the noise suppression seems to be negligible. This is also reflected in the high standard deviations of the noise standard deviation between the different image regions in Tab. 8.1. In average, a noise reduction rate of about 38% was achieved, but with a standard deviation of about 10%. The same effect is visible in the values of the SNR-gain. In comparison to a linear filter some regions are filtered much stronger than others. From the variation of the standard deviations of noise within the different pixel regions it is visible, that although in average the noise was reduced, e. g. from 20.5 HU to 13.3 HU, the variation between the regions kept about the same or even slightly increased from 6.4 HU to 6.9 HU. Compared to the mean noise the variation of noise over the image domain was even increased.

In contrast to that, the proposed adaptive bilateral filter reduces the amount of noise in the image, but also the variation between the different pixel regions. This can be seen for both configurations of the proposed filter, also from the example images shown in Fig. 8.4(c) and Fig. 8.4(d). In average, the standard deviation of noise was reduced about 24% with $r = 1$ and 56% with $r = 2$, with only a low variation between the different pixel regions of 1.4-2.4%. Regarding the SNR-gain, the proposed method shows much lower variation between the different pixel regions than the standard bilateral filter. With respect to a noise-resolution-tradeoff, the computed values for the SNR-gain show that in nearly all cases the resolution was preserved well. In comparison to a simple linear filtering that leads to the same smoothing at the edge the NABF methods show a clear advantag. Only for very low contrast-to-noise levels around 1 the edges can no longer be differentiated from noise and thus the SNR-gain clearly drops. At contrast-to-noise levels between 3 to 5 the noise reduction can already be seen as a real gain, because the SNR-gain is close to the NRR.

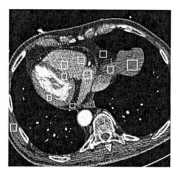

(a) Original

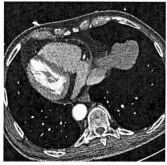

(b) Noise-adaptive bilateral filter

(c) Standard bilateral filter

Figure 8.6: Clinically acquired thorax scan. Comparison of standard bilateral filter and noise adaptive bilateral filter.

8.4.2 Example Images

In Fig. 8.6 an example of a clinically acquired thorax scan is shown. The standard deviation of noise was evaluated in 10 pixel regions, as illustrated in the noisy original slice shown in Fig. 8.6(a). The standard deviation of noise in the original image of 72.0 ± 14.5 HU was reduced to 48.0 ± 15.9 HU for the SBF and to 44.4 ± 9.9 HU with our proposed NABF. Here it can again be observed that the proposed NABF reduces the standard deviation of noise and noise between the different pixel regions becomes more homogeneous. The SBF, on the other hand, assumes all pixel values in the image are equally reliable. Therefore, some regions in the image are smoothed stronger than others. At the end this results in a noise suppressed image, too, but the standard deviation between the noise standard deviations in the different pixel regions even increased.

8.5 Conclusions

In this chapter a new approach for computing orientation dependent noise estimates was presented. Based on the theory of the Fourier-Slice theorem, the direction, which mostly contributes to the local noise variance during backprojection can be determined for each image pixel. The overall noise variance can then be split up into its contribution along and orthogonal to this direction. With this technique it is possible to obtain information about the local noise correlation in the image without evaluating the complete covariance matrix. The additional information about local noise variance and correlation can be used for adapting post-processing methods to the non-stationary and non-isotropic noise in the reconstructed image. The effectiveness was demonstrated on the example of a bilateral filter. The evaluation on simulated and clinically acquired data showed that a noise reduction close to 60% could be achieved without noticable loss of resolution. Only for contrasts very close to the noise level, the edges can no longer be perfectly preserved. For CNR levels larger than 3 the noise reduction rate can already be seen as a real gain in SNR, because the perforance of the NABF is improved with respect to noise recution at the same average resolution, compared to a simple linear filtering.

Chapter 9

Discussion

The non-stationary and non-isotropic noise in reconstructed CT datasets makes the use of specially adapted methods for noise reduction indispensable. In the previous chapters, basically two different approaches for noise adaptive filtering of CT reconstructions were introduced. In the first part of this work, wavelet based noise reduction methods were discussed, which use two input datasets. Correlation analysis between the wavelet representations of the two input datasets and noise estimation in the wavelet domain is used for differentiating between structure and noise. In the second part, noise is analyzed in the measured projection data. The propagation of variances and covariances through the reconstruction algorithm gives an estimate of the local image noise. The estimated local noise variance and noise correlation is then used for noise adaptive filtering.

The evaluation of the different approaches already showed that high noise reduction rates of about 60% can be achieved with both approaches, while anatomical structures are well preserved. In this chapter the different proposed noise reduction methods are compared to each other. The visual appearance of the processed datasets, as well as quantitative criteria like noise reduction and resolution are considered. Based on the analysis of noise and resolution, the potential for dose reduction is discussed. Furthermore, the computational requirements of the different approaches are analyzed and possible optimizations are discussed. After the comparison of the methods, possible directions for future work are considered.

9.1 Comparison of Proposed Noise Reduction Methods

If noise reduction methods for the use in CT are compared, different aspects are of interest. First of all, the visual appearance of the processed data plays an important role. Especially, if the noise suppressed data should not just be used for post-processing applications. The processed images or volumes used for diagnosis should ideally look like CT images acquired at a higher radiation dose. Noise in the images should be reduced, but resolution ideally be preserved. Furthermore, it is important that the images are free of artifacts and do not strongly change the noise pattern. Important for the comparison of noise reduction methods is of course also the quantitative comparison. If non-linear filtering techniques are applied, resolution at the edges changes depending on the contrast of the edge. Consequently, a contrast dependent analysis of the noise reduction methods needs to be performed. The noise reduction performance of a certain algorithm should always be considered together with the influence on image resolution. With respect to practical usability of the proposed algorithms not only the image quality plays an important role. The computational efficiency of the algorithms is also worth of consideration. Therefore, the computational and storage costs of the certain algorithms are analyzed and discussed.

The above described aspects are in the following compared between the wavelet based noise reduction method, described in Chapter 6, and the noise-adaptive bilateral filtering introduced in Chapter 8. The qualitative, as well as the quantitative comparison is done based on the same simulated CT datasets. The elliptical water phantom, described in Section 6.4, with a cylindrical inlay of varying contrasts is used.

9.1.1 Qualitative Comparison

In Fig. 9.1 one example of a noisy slice together with the results of the noise-adaptive bilateral filtering at two different denoising strengths ($r = 1.0$ and $r = 2.0$) is shown. The different wavelet based denoising techniques applied to the same example slice can be found in Fig. 9.2. The wavelet filtering results are shown for different wavelet transformations, the 2-D-DWT, 2-D-SWT and 3-D-DWT all in combination with a simple Haar wavelet. Two different filtering strengths are compared here ($p = 1.0$ and $p = 2.0$).

The following observations can be made by visual inspection:

- The 2-D-DWT in combination with Haar wavelet tends to show visible blocky regions in the noise suppressed image. Especially, in case of stronger noise suppression like in Fig. 9.2(b), the processed images show strange noise patterns and are no longer suitable for diagnostic imaging.

- The blocky regions that are visible with 2-D-DWT can be eliminated by using the redundant and shift-invariant wavelet transformation 2-D-SWT instead. The noise suppressed images in Fig. 9.2(c) and Fig. 9.2(d) look more natural.

- Clearly, best results with respect to noise reduction and preservation of edges are obtained with the 3-D-DWT. The images look very natural with respect to the remaining noise in the image, even in case of stronger noise suppression, like in Fig. 9.2(f).

- In comparison to the wavelet approaches, the NABF approach which is just working on 2-D datasets, shows good results. The original noise pattern seems not strongly changed, just reduced in its amplitude.

9.1.2 Noise and Resolution

The influence of the different denoising approaches to noise and resolution has already been discussed in detail at the end of each chapter. Here the main observations are summarized and the wavelet based approaches are compared to the noise-adaptive bilateral filtering. The comparison between several noise reduction methods is not an easy task. A fair comparison is only possible if image noise is evaluated at the same image resolution. Achieving the same image resolution for all approaches, on the other hand, is nearly impossible. At least if non-linear methods are applied to the images, image resolution might differ between the different image regions, and, as already shown in the evaluation

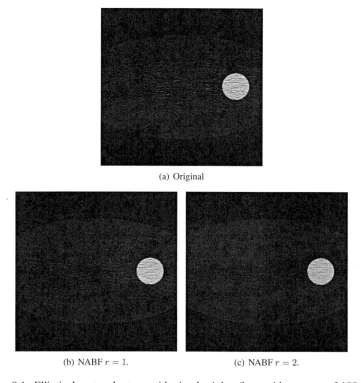

(a) Original

(b) NABF $r = 1$.

(c) NABF $r = 2$.

Figure 9.1: Elliptical water phantom with circular inlay (here with contrast of 100 HU). Original noisy slice and noise-adaptive bilateral filtered images (NABF) with two different strengths of noise suppression ($r = 1$ and $r = 2$). Display: c=50, w=200.

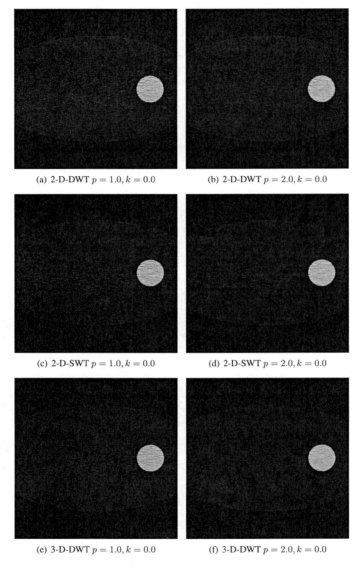

(a) 2-D-DWT $p = 1.0, k = 0.0$ (b) 2-D-DWT $p = 2.0, k = 0.0$

(c) 2-D-SWT $p = 1.0, k = 0.0$ (d) 2-D-SWT $p = 2.0, k = 0.0$

(e) 3-D-DWT $p = 1.0, k = 0.0$ (f) 3-D-DWT $p = 2.0, k = 0.0$

Figure 9.2: Elliptical water phantom with circular inlay (here with contrast of 100 HU). Wavelet based noise reduction method with different wavelet transformations (2-D-DWT, 2-D-SWT, 3-D-DWT) and different strengths of noise suppression ($p = 1.0$ and $p = 2.0$), without using significance weighting ($k = 0.0$). Display: c=50, w=200.

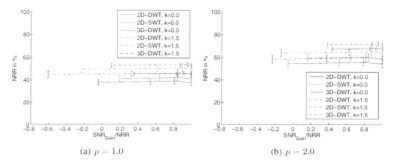

(a) $p = 1.0$ (b) $p = 2.0$

Figure 9.3: Noise-Resolution-Tradeoff - Comparison of NRR for different values of p without ($k = 0.0$ solid) and with ($k = 1.5$ dashed) significance weights in combination with different wavelet transformations 2-D-DWT (blue), 2-D-SWT (gray) and 3-D-DWT (red).

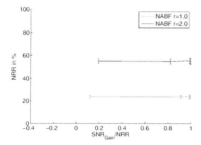

Figure 9.4: Noise-Resolution-Tradeoff - NABF with two different noise suppression strengths ($r = 1.0$ and $r = 2.0$).

sections of the previous chapters, also at differently contrasted edges. In addition to the noise-reduction rate (NRR in Eq. (6.9)), a new figure of merit, the SNR-gain (SNRG in Eq. (6.10)), has already been introduced in Chapter 6 for measuring the noise-resolution-tradeoff.

The main idea of the evaluation strategy is briefly summarized here. The local average MTF at the edge of a circular inlay is computed. From the MTF measured in the original image and the MTF in the processed image, a linear filter can be computed, which leads to the average same smoothing at the edge. The linear filter is then also applied to the noisy image. The standard deviation of noise in different pixel regions (here 12 different regions) is than compared to the standard deviation of noise in the original image (giving the NRR defined in Eq. (6.9)) and to the standard deviation in the linearly filtered image (giving the SNRG defined in Eq. (6.10)). The quotient of NRR and SNRG is then used as a measurement for the edge-preservation capability of the method. It measures how much the adaptive filtering can be seen as a gain compared to a simple linear filtering that leads to the same average smoothing at the edge. If a quotient close to 1 is obtained, the edge at the circular inlay was perfectly preserved and the noise reduction can be seen as a real gain. Otherwise, if the ratio is below 1, this means that the edge was not perfectly preserved. The edge was smoothed and consequently, the linear filter that leads to the same average smoothing at the edge performed like a lowpass filter.

The NRR and the ratio between SNRG and NRR is plotted in Fig. 9.4 for the NABF and in Fig. 9.3 for the wavelet based approaches. Each line line in the plot consists of four points. They correspond to the evaluations at the four different contrast-to-noise levels that were considered. The contrast at the circular inlay compared to water was varied between 20, 60, 100 and 1000 HU. Accordingly, the CNR at the edge of the inlay varied between 1, 3, 5 and 50. It can be seen clearly, that for all different noise reduction approaches the resolution was perfectly preserved, because the ratio between SNRG and NRR is close to 1. The noise reduction rate can thus be seen as a real gain. With decreasing contrast, the edges are no longer perfectly detected and get smoothed. The lower the contrast at the edge, the stronger this effect is noticeable.

If we compare the different approaches, it can be observed that for the wavelet based filtering methods the performance differs between the different wavelet transformation methods. The 2-D-SWT is better than 2-D-DWT and 3-D-DWT is better than both 2-D transformations. This observation holds for the NRR as well as for the edge-preservation capability. Furthermore, it can be seen that higher NRR can be achieved if significance weights ($k = 1.5$) are used compared to no significance weights ($k = 0.0$). For very low contrasts, however the preservation of edges is slightly reduced, using significance weights. With $p = 1.0$ lower noise reduction of around 37-54% is achieved than for $p = 2.0$, which results in NRR of about 54-73%.

The NRR obtained with the NABF is about 24% for $r = 1.0$ and 55% for $r = 2.0$. In comparison to the wavelet based noise reduction approaches, the edge-preservation with the bilateral filter is better. Even for a CNR of 5 the edge is nearly not smoothed and the SNRG/NRR is close to one. For lower CNR around 1 SNR without significance weighting is comparable to the NABF. The 3-D-DWT based filtering is even better than the NABF, in both NRR and edge-preservation.

9.1.3   Potential for Dose Reduction

The close relation between the radiation dose used for the acquisition of the projections and the noise in the reconstructed CT datasets has already been pointed out in Section 2.4. The standard deviation of noise in the reconstructed image is indirectly proportional to the square root of the dose D [Kale 00]:

$$\sigma \propto \frac{1}{\sqrt{D}}, \tag{9.1}$$

which holds as long as quantum noise is the most dominant source of noise and other effects, like electronic noise, are negligible. Goal of the noise reduction methods proposed in this thesis is either:

- Improving the signal-to-noise ratio in the image without increasing the radiation dose, or

- Decreasing the radiation dose without decreasing the signal-to-noise ratio.

The amount of noise reduction and the associated influence on image resolution as been discussed in detail in the last section. In this section we will now concentrate on the analysis of the potential of dose reduction. More precisely, we are interested in how strong the radiation dose can be decreased, such that in combination with one of the proposed noise reduction methods no loss of image quality is noticeable compared to the image obtained at the common dose. Image quality is here only considered with respect to the standard deviation of noise and spatial resolution.

In a first step, we consider the upper limit of dose reduction based on the achieved reduction of the standard deviation of noise in the image. For the moment we do not take into account the influence on image resolution. According to the proportionality expressed in Eq. (9.1) the following holds:

$$\frac{D_{\min}}{D_{\text{orig}}} = \frac{\sigma_{\text{afil}}^2}{\sigma_{\text{orig}}^2},\tag{9.2}$$

where σ_{afil}^2 is the standard deviation of noise in the adaptively filtered image (using one of the proposed noise reduction methods), σ_{orig}^2 is the standard deviation of noise in the original image. The dose D_{orig} was used for the acquisition of the original image and $D_{\min}$ corresponds to the dose that would be necessary to acquire an image with standard deviation σ_{afil}^2 without using an adaptive filter. The upper limit for dose reduction rate $\text{DRR}_{\max}$ can, thus, be defined as:

$$\text{DRR}_{\max} = 1 - \frac{D_{\min}}{D_{\text{orig}}} = 1 - \frac{\sigma_{\text{afil}}^2}{\sigma_{\text{orig}}^2} = 1 - (1 - \text{NRR})^2.\tag{9.3}$$

If we now take the noise reduction rates from the last section, we obtain that the NRR of 37-54% of the wavelet based filter with $p = 1.0$ corresponds to a $\text{DRR}_{\max}$ of 60-79%, and the NRR of 54-73% for $p = 2.0$ corresponds to a $\text{DRR}_{\max}$ of 79-93%. In case of the NABF we get a $\text{DRR}_{\max}$ of 42% for $r = 1.0$ and 80% for $r = 2.0$.

The analysis presented so far does not take into account the resolution in the processed images. If we only consider the $\text{DRR}_{\max}$ for a filter, arbitrarily high dose reduction rates could also be achieved with linear filters. However, structures in the image get blurred and the low dose acquisition using $D_{\min}$ with the applied post-processing filter is clearly not comparable with the unprocessed image acquired at the original dose D_{orig}. Only if the edges in the image are not influenced in image resolution in the processed image, the maximum dose reduction rate is really achievable. The investigation of the noise-resolution-tradeoff in the previous section showed that the smoothing of edges, due to the application of the proposed algorithms, depends on the CNR at the edge. It must be taken into account that the CNR at the edge in the low dose acquisition (CNR_{low}) is reduced compared to the CNR in the original image (CNR_{orig}):

$$\text{CNR}_{\text{low}} = \sqrt{D_{\min}/D_{\text{orig}}}\,\text{CNR}_{\text{orig}} = \sqrt{1 - \text{DRR}_{\max}}\,\text{CNR}_{\text{orig}},\tag{9.4}$$

because the noise in the low dose acquisition is increased. We then get a more realistic approximation of the achievable dose reduction rate on the basis of the SNR-gain, evaluated at an edge with CNR_{low}, according to:

$$\text{DRR}_{\text{app}} = \begin{cases} 1 - (1 - \text{SNRG})^2 & \text{if} \quad \text{SNRG} > 0 \\ 0 & \text{otherwise} \end{cases}.\tag{9.5}$$

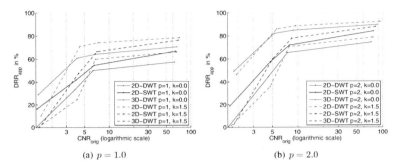

(a) $p = 1.0$ (b) $p = 2.0$

Figure 9.5: Potential for dose reduction of wavelet based noise reduction methods - Comparison of $\mathrm{DRR_{app}}$ for different values of p without ($k = 0.0$ solid) and with ($k = 1.5$ dashed) significance weights in combination with different wavelet transformations 2-D-DWT (blue), 2-D-SWT (gray) and 3-D-DWT (red).

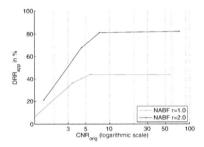

Figure 9.6: Potential for dose reduction of noise adaptive bilateral filter - Comparison of $\mathrm{DRR_{app}}$ for NABF with two different noise suppression strengths ($r = 1.0$ and $r = 2.0$).

This approximation of the achievable dose reduction rate takes into account the loss of resolution due to the filtering. If no resolution was lost at the edge the SNRG is equivalent to the NRR and $\mathrm{DRR_{app}} = \mathrm{DRR_{max}}$. Otherwise, $\mathrm{DRR_{app}} < \mathrm{DRR_{max}}$ depending on the ratio between SNRG and NRR.

The estimated potential for dose reduction of the wavelet based denoising approaches are presented in Fig. 9.5. In Fig. 9.6 the estimated dose reduction rates are shown for the NABF. The $\mathrm{DRR_{app}}$ values, computed according to Eq. (9.5), are plotted against the CNR in the original images. From the plots it can be seen that the expected potential for dose reduction varies depending on the minimum CNR level we are interested in in the original image. Consequently, it depends on the clinical application how much dose can be saved by applying one of the proposed post-processing filters. If very low contrasts close to CNR values of 1 are of interest for the application, there is no or only low potential for dose reduction, because it is difficult to preserve structures at very low contrasts in image acquired at a lower dose. But even for low CNR levels between 3 to 5 the application of the proposed filters to low dose images can lead to a noticeable reduction of radiation dose up to 60% in 2-D and even close to 80% in 3-D. For CNR levels higher than 5 there is not much difference in the estimated dose reduction compared to very high CNR levels around 50, because edges with a CNR of about 5 can already be well preserved.

9.1.4 Computational Performance

Although noise reduction methods are usually seen as post-processing methods, the here presented approaches are not simply applied to a reconstructed CT dataset as one would expect for a typical post-processing application. Both algorithms require the acquired CT projection data. The wavelet based approach for reconstructing two volumes from disjoint subsets of projections, the noise-adaptive bilateral filtering for performing the noise propagation through the reconstruction algorithm. In both cases special processing of the projection data is necessary for generating the required input data for the noise reduction algorithms. The computational requirements for generating the input data is, thus, the first thing to be analyzed. After that the computational complexity of the noise reduction algorithms themselves are analyzed.

Generation of Input Datasets

As already mentioned before, the wavelet method requires two input datasets. Different possibilities for generating two input datasets are described in Section 4.2. It is possible to use successive scans, split up one acquisition into even and odd numbered projections, or use a dual-source CT-scanner. If two successive scans are used, two complete reconstructions need to be performed. If one acquisition is split up into two disjoint subsets of projections, two reconstruction, but both at only half the number of projections is required. It is however, important to notice that only if a linear reconstruction algorithm is used, the sum of the two separate reconstructions is equivalent to the reconstruction from the complete number of projections. Otherwise, it is better to additionally compute the reconstruction from the complete set of projections and apply the computed weights to its wavelet coefficients. The acquisition with a dual-source CT directly results in two projection datasets. The projections acquired at the one detector are used for the reconstruction of the first, the projections acquired at the other detector for the reconstruction of the second input dataset. Altogether, it can be summarized that all different approaches for generating the two input datasets require two complete reconstructions.

The noise-adaptive bilateral filtering takes just one reconstructed CT dataset as its input. Additionally, it requires the variance map that shows for each image pixel an estimate of the local noise variance. Furthermore, the orientation dependent variance map is needed, which shows a pixel wise estimate of the variance contribution of a certain orientation, e.g. in direction of the strongest correlation, to the overall noise variance. This orientation dependent variance map gives information about the local noise correlation and consequently, the noise-anisotropy. The computation of the variance maps is based on the noise propagation algorithm described in Chapter 7. It is basically another reconstruction, however, a modified reconstruction that allows the computation of noise variances. The computational performance of the noise propagation method is comparable with the reconstruction of the HU-values. Nevertheless, more computations are involved due to the correlation estimations during the noise propagation. The computation of the variance map and the orientation dependent variance map can partially be performed together. They only differ in the backprojection step. Here, it is necessary to first compute the backprojection loop for the variance map, where at the same time the direction of strongest correlation is determined. The direction of strongest correlation is obtained by detecting for each image pixel the projection angle from which the strongest contribution to the overall noise variance is achieved. In a second backprojection loop the weighted backprojection of the noise variance is computed based on the pixelwise determined direction of strongest correlation. In sum one and a half additional reconstructions of noise variances need to be performed in addition to the standard reconstruction of the HU-values.

Noise Reduction Algorithm

After the generation of the input datasets the main part of the method, the noise reduction algorithm can start. The core of the wavelet based approaches is the computation of the wavelet representation of the input datasets. As already described above, the wavelet denoising techniques presented here require two input datasets, which are both decomposed into its wavelet coefficients. Different wavelet transformations can be used for this decomposition. As the above discussion showed, the 2-D-SWT outperforms the 2-D-DWT and the best visual and quantitative results are achieved with the 3-D-DWT. The use of the stationary wavelet transformation, on the one hand, or the three-dimensional transformation, on the other hand, do not only come with better denoising results, but also with increased computational and storage cost. While one decomposition step of the 2-D-DWT has a complexity of $O(N \log N)$ for an image of $N \times N$ pixels, the 2-D-SWT has a complexity of $O(N^2)$. The SWT, furthermore, does not perform a downsampling step after the filtering and consequently, the number of pixels in the approximation image is constant over all the decomposition levels, meaning that for all levels l up to the maximum decomposition level the same number of computations needs to be performed. The downsampling of the DWT reduces size of the approximation image at level l to $2^{-l}N \times 2^{-l}N$ and accordingly fewer computations are necessary for the decomposition at level $l + 1$. The 3-D-DWT has a complexity of $O(N \log N \log \log N)$ for a volume of N^3 pixels, where the number of coefficients is kept constant, regardless of the maximum decomposition level.

Especially, for the further processing on the basis of the wavelet representation of the input data, it plays an important role, if a downsampling step is performed or not. For each detail coefficient of the wavelet representation an according weight needs to be computed, in order to suppress the noisy coefficients. The number of computations scales with the number of detail coefficients. The number of detail coefficients up to the maximum decomposition level $l_{\max}$ in case of DWT amounts to $3 \sum_{l=1}^{l_{\max}} (2^{-l}N)^2$. In case of 2-D-SWT the number of overall detail coefficients is $3l_{\max}N^2$, and for 3-D-DWT we have $7 \sum_{l=1}^{l_{\max}} (2^{-l}N)^3$. The respective weights can be computed efficiently and only small local neighborhoods are needed. The weights are computed independently for each detail coefficient, which means that this step can be well be parallelized, or computed on streaming architecture, like graphics cards.

After the weighting of the detail coefficients one inverse wavelet transformation is necessary. The computational cost of an inverse DWT is comparable with the DWT decomposition. The inverse SWT, however, is computational more expensive, if the redundancy of the data should ideally be used for the reconstruction. Depending on the redundancy factor

R at a respective decomposition level, R times the computations of an inverse DWT are necessary. The redundancy at level l of the SWT is $R = 2^l$.

The noise-adaptive bilateral filtering can be computed in $O(N^2)$. For each image pixel a weighted sum with its local neighborhood is computed for determining the noise suppressed new pixel value. All pixels can be calculated independently. The algorithm is, thus, well suited for parallel computing.

9.2 Suggestions for Future Research

The application of edge-preserving filters to reconstructed CT images is a relatively new approach and is so far not commonly applied in clinical practice. The examinations of the previous section showed the practical applicability of the proposed algorithms and demonstrated that potentially a remarkable gain in signal-to-noise ratio can be achieved with the new techniques. Nevertheless, some open questions and possibilities for further improvements remain. It has been shown that with better knowledge about the local noise properties in the reconstructed datasets improved noise-adaptive filtering methods can be developed. The deeper investigation of methods for noise analysis, also in 3D, is thus an important part for future research. Furthermore, the use of other sparse representations like the curvelet transformation, can potentially lead to improvements in noise reduction in CT. In the following some ideas for future research are described.

9.2.1 Noise Analysis Methods

Throughout this thesis, it has been shown that one of the keys for the development of efficacious noise reduction methods is to have precise knowledge about the underlying noise characteristics. In CT, noise in the acquired projection data can be well described by physical models. The noise in the projections then propagates through the reconstruction algorithm to the reconstructed volumes. Noise in the images is thus a direct result of the noise in the measurements, but can no longer be easily described. It is necessary to use noise propagation algorithms in order to determine the local noise variance and correlation. Such noise propagation algorithms might become rather complicated and computational expensive, especially, if all correlations of the input data or induced during the processing should be taken into account. The proposed approximation scheme for estimating the correlation within the data based on linear system theory, as introduced in chapter Chapter 7 might also be applicable in the context of other reconstruction methods. In this thesis, the noise propagation has only been investigated for 2-D indirect fan-beam FBP reconstruction. The application of the here presented theory in 3-D reconstruction methods, like the weighted filtered backprojection (WFBP), is one field for future research.

Another interesting aspect is the frequency dependent analysis of the noise after reconstruction. Some post-processing methods, like the wavelet based noise reduction, decompose the reconstructions into frequency bands and process on the frequency representation of the data. For this purpose, it would be beneficial to have access to the noise variance and correlation in the respective frequency band. It is possible to perform a frequency selection during reconstruction, for example by modifying the reconstruction kernel, e. g. by multiplying its frequency response with a bandpass filter. If the noise propagation is then performed with the modified reconstruction kernel the noise variance can be computed for a certain frequency band. An interesting investigation would be to compare if this more precise frequency dependent noise analysis helps in improving the noise reduction algorithms. It might also be possible to compute the noise in the wavelet coefficients of the reconstructed dataset directly from the noise estimates in the projections. Here, the theory on multiresolution reconstruction [Dela 95, Bonn 02] might be helpful for developing noise estimation methods for wavelet coefficients of reconstructed CT datasets.

9.2.2   Noise Reduction in CT

The evaluation of the different proposed noise reduction methods already showed, that noise reduction in 3-D gives best results with respect to noise reduction and preservation of structures. So far the NABF has only been considered in 2-D, because methods for noise propagation of 3-D reconstruction methods, like the WFBP are so far not available. Based on the comparison between the 2-D wavelet based noise reduction and the NABF it could be observed that improved edge-preservation at comparable NRR is achieved with NABF. It is, therefore, promising to obtain even better results by extending the noise propagation and NABF to 3-D.

Of course, the computed variance and orientation dependent contributions to the noise variance that were proposed in this thesis, can potentially be used for adapting other postprocessing methods to the non-stationary and non-isotropic noise in reconstructed CT datasets. Other filtering methods, or image processing techniques like segmentation and registration could make use of the knowledge about the noise statistics in the image or volume. Especially, for methods, which are based on image gradients, it would be helpful to have an estimate of the uncertainty of the reconstructed image pixels, in order to differentiate between gradients that are computed due to noise or real structures.

Another idea for future research would be to use other sparse representations, like the curvelet transformation [Star 02] for noise reduction in CT. It combines the resolution hierarchy known from wavelet transformations and the Radon transformation and is thus closely related to CT reconstruction. Noise reduction in the projection domain has the advantage of having good estimates of the noise variance. The Signal-to-noise ratio is, however, better after reconstruction, because during the backprojection process an averaging of many noisy samples is performed. In this work the combination of both advantages was performed by estimating noise in the reconstructed dataset from the projections and use this for noise reduction. Based on the curvelet transformation the good knowledge about the noise statistics in the projection data and the good localization of edges in the reconstructed data can be combined. It is however necessary, to include noise estimation approaches for curvelet based noise reduction in CT. So far the proposed thresholding approaches only consider white Gaussian noise in the reconstructed images. The noise propagation approach introduced in this thesis could also be used for improved threshold determination of the curvelet coefficients of a CT dataset. Furthermore, the extension of the curvelet transformation to 3-D is still under investigation and could probably be more closely investigated in the context of 3-D reconstruction.

Chapter 10

Summary and Conclusions

In this thesis methods for structure-preserving noise reduction in reconstructed CT datasets were investigated. The goal was to improve the signal-to-noise ratio without increasing the radiation dose or noticeably affecting the spatial resolution. Due to the close relation between image noise and radiation dose, this improvement at the same time opens up a possibility for dose reduction. Two different original approaches for noise reduction in CT were developed, implemented and evaluated.

The first part of the thesis covers wavelet based noise reduction methods. They are based on the idea of using reconstructions from two disjoint subsets of projections as input to the noise reduction algorithm. The two input datasets are generated such that they show the same structure, but differ with respect to noise. Correlation analysis between the wavelet coefficients of the two input datasets can then be used for differentiating between structure and noise. We evaluated the proposed method in combination with different wavelet transformation techniques with respect to noise and resolution. It turned out, that the non-redundant SWT showed best qualitative and quantitative results. High noise reduction rates about 45% were achieved. Within a human observer study the low-contrast-detectability was evaluated. The experiment showed that even small objects with a contrast-to-noise level close to 1 can be detected as good, or even better after the application of the adaptive filter in comparison to the unmodified original image. The comparison with a state-of-the-art projection based noise reduction method, furthermore, showed that better edge-preservation at comparable noise reduction is obtained with the new method. In order to allow anisotropic filtering in the wavelet domain, a technique for noise estimation from the difference of the two input datasets was proposed. The comparison of the computed noise estimates with results from Monte-Carlo showed that average pixelwise relative errors between 11.6% and 20.7% are achieved. A noise estimation based on just two measurements, thus only allows a rough estimation of the pixelwise standard deviation of noise. Nevertheless, the proposed thresholding method based on local, frequency and orientation dependent noise estimates leads to an anisotropic filtering and shows much better results than standard wavelet thresholding methods in case of CT. Especially, for datasets with strongly directed noise, like in the shoulders or hips, improved results are obtained with the proposed algorithm. We then combined the correlation analysis and noise estimation and extended the algorithm to 3-D. The noise reduction in 3-D showed much better results than in 2-D. The processed images look more natural in case of 3-D. Furthermore, higher noise reduction rates of more than 60% are obtained.

In the second part of the thesis, a new approach that is based on noise propagation through the reconstruction algorithm was introduced. The noise variance in the reconstructed image is a direct result of noise in the projections. We developed an original approach for computing pixelwise estimates of the noise variance in the image reconstructed with indirect fan-beam FBF. The difficulty is that the rebinning step, which reorganizes the acquired fan-beam projections to parallel-beam projections, correlates the data. In contrast to other approaches the correlations introduced to the data during the reconstruction are modeled by linear system theory and are taken into account. With the new noise propagation method average pixelwise relative errors between 2.0% and 6.7% are achieved. The noise propagation approach was then extended in order to additionally give information about the local noise correlation. We proposed a sine-/cosine-square-weighting of the noise variances in the projections and separate noise propagation in order to obtain the horizontal and vertical contribution of the noise variance for every pixel. The approach was then improved such that for each individual pixel a specific separation into two orthogonal directions can be computed. The variance contribution in direction of strongest correlation and orthogonal to that can be determined for each pixel. This additional knowledge was then used for developing noise-adaptive filtering methods. We proposed a bilateral filter, which adapts itself to the non-stationary and non-isotropic noise in CT. With this method noise reduction rates close to 60% were achieved in 2-D.

In addition to the development of new noise reduction methods for CT, this work also presented some new ideas for the evaluation of non-linear filters. Clearly, the reduction of the noise variance in the image is an important quality criteria, but the influence on the spatial resolution plays an important role, too. Usually, spatial resolution is only considered at high contrast objects. If non-linear processing is performed, image resolution might change depending on the local contrast-to-noise ratio. Therefore, a contrast dependent evaluation of the spatial resolution was introduced. Furthermore, we proposed a new figure of merit for the noise-resolution-tradeoff, we call SNR-gain. The evaluation is based on the comparison to the linear filter, which leads to the same average spatial resolution. The new evaluation method can be used for more realistically judging the potential for dose reduction, depending on the clinical task. The estimated dose reduction rates that were computed on basis of the new noise-resolution-tradeoff do not simply consider the improvement of image noise by the application of the filter. They also consider the loss of resolution at a certain contrast-to-noise ratio. Depending on the clinical application, the minimum contrasts that are of interest might vary. If lesions should be detected very low contrasts are usually of interest, on the contrary, in case of bone fractures very high contrasts are of interest. If very low contrasts close to CNR values of 1 need to be differentiated, there is no or only low potential for dose reduction, because it is difficult to preserve structures at very low contrasts in image acquired at a lower dose. Based on our proposed estimation of the potential for dose reduction we can conclude that even for low CNR levels between 3 to 5 the application of the proposed filters to low dose images can lead to a noticeable reduction of radiation dose up to 60% in 2-D and even close to 80% in 3-D. It should, however, be reminded that an extended clinical study is necessary to proove these estimates in clinical practice also in context of different diagnostic and treatment assesment tasks.

Appendix A

Acronyms

A.1 CT Reconstruction

CT   computed tomography
MSCT   mulit-slice computed tomography
DSCT   dual-source computed tomography
FBP   filtered backprojection
WFBP   weighted filtered backprojection
SMP   segmented multiple plane
HU   Hounsfield Unit
FOV   field of view
MTF   modulation transfer function
SNR   signal-to-noise ratio
CNR   contrast-to-noise ratio
PSF   point-spread-function
LSF   line-spread-function
lp   line-pairs

A.2 Wavelet Transformation

WT   wavelet transformation
CWT   continuous wavelet transformation
WFT   windowed Fourier transformation
STFT   short-time Fourier transformation
DWT   discrete time wavelet transformation
SWT   shift-invariant wavelet transformation
ATR   á-trous wavelet transformation
FFT   fast Fourier transformation
Db2   Daubechies 2 wavelet
CDF9/7 Cohen-Daubechies-Fauraune wavelet

A.3   Denoising

CORR	correlation coefficient based weighting
GRAD	gradient approximation based weighting
S80	sharp reconstruction kernel
B40	smoother reconstruction kernel
ROC	receiver operating characteristic
TPR	true positive rate
FPR	false positive rate
STSWT	standard thresholding using on SWT
ANESWT	adaptive noise-estimation based thresholding using SWT
CASWT	correlation based weighting using SWT
NRR	noise reduction rate
SNRG	SNR-gain
SBF	standard bilateral filtering
NABF	noise-adaptive bilateral filtering

A.4   Noise Propagation

ACF	auto correlation function
ACCF	auto correlation coefficient function
WSS	wide sense stationary

Appendix B

Notation

B.1 CT Reconstruction

I_0	intesity at source
N_0	number of emitted photons at source
I	intesity at detector
r	focus radius
α	focus angle
β	fan angle
θ	parallel projection angle
t	orthogonal distance to iso-center
L	ray
$\mathbf{x}$	2-D or 3-D spatial position
x, y, z	spatial coordinates
P	projection
$P(\alpha, \beta)$	fan-beam projection
$P(\theta, t)$	parallel-beam projection
$\mathcal{F}$	Fourier transformation operator
$\mathcal{R}$	Radon transformation operator
μ	attenuation coefficient
μ_w	attenuation coefficient of water
k_r	ramp kernel
k	apodized convolution kernel
q	apodization window
μ	attenuation coefficient
μ_w	attenuation coefficient of water

N_f	number of channels in fan-beam projection
$N_{2\pi f}$	number of fan-beam projections in 2π
N_p	number of channels in parallel projection
$N_{2\pi p}$	number of parallel projections in 2π
$N_{\pi p}$	number of parallel projections in π
$\Delta\alpha, \Delta\beta, \ldots$	sampling distances/ increments
$k, l \ldots$	indices
$P_{k,l}^{fan}$	fan-beam projection at α_k and β_l
$P_{m,l}^{hyb}$	hybrid projection at θ_m and β_l
$P_{i,j}^{com}$	complementary rebinned projection at θ_i and β_j
$P_{i,n}^{par}$	parallel-beam projection at θ_i and t_n
$\overset{*}{P}_{i,n}^{par}$	filtered parallel-beam projection
h	interpolation function
h^{azi}	azimuthal interpolation function
h^{rad}	radial interpolation function
h^{bpj}	backprojection interpolation function
f	function to be reconstructed in HU
$\mathbf{x}$	Cartesian coordinates, position
U	signal measured at detector
N_U	measurement error/noise of signal
N_q	quantum noise
N_e	electronics noise
$c, \tilde{c}$	constants
n	number of X-ray quanta quanta
$\mathcal{P}$	probability distribution
$\mathcal{E}$	expectation
σ_q^2	variance of quantum noise
σ_e^2	variance of electronics noise
σ_I^2	variance of intensity
σ_P^2	variance of projection
W	highest spatial frequency within measured projection

B.2 Wavelet Transformation

f	function
w	window function
w^*	complex conjugate of w
ψ	wavelet function (mother wavelet)
ϕ	scaling function (father wavelet)
s	scaling factor
τ	translation
Ψ	Fourier representation of ψ
s_j	dyadic scale
τ_k	translation corresponding to dyadic scale
j, k	indices
$d_{j,k}$	detail coefficient at scale s_j and translation τ_k
$c_{j,k}$	approximation coefficient at scale s_j and translation τ_k
g	analysis lowpass filter
h	analysis highpass filter
$\tilde{g}$	synthesis lowpass filter
$\tilde{h}$	synthesis highpass filter
$A = A_0$	image (approximation at level 0)
$s = 2^{-J}$	scale of input image
l	decomposition level
$l_{\max}$	maximum decomposition level
A_l	approximation at level l
$W_{A,l}^{\mathrm{H}}$	horizontal detail coefficient of A at level l
$W_{A,l}^{\mathrm{V}}$	vertical detail coefficient of A at level l
$W_{A,l}^{\mathrm{D}}$	diagonal detail coefficient of A at level l
$g_l, h_l, \tilde{g}_l, \tilde{h}_l$	analysis and synthesis filters used at level l
$G, H, \tilde{G}_l, \tilde{H}_l$	z-transformations of filters

B.3   Wavelet Denoising

A, B	input datasets (2D, 3D)
P	set of projections
P1	first subset of projections
P2	second subset of projections
P_i	projections at angle θ_i
$\mathcal{R}^\star$	reconstruction operator
M	mean of input datasets / reconstruction from all projections
D	difference of input datasets
S	noise-free signal
N	zero-mean additive noise
$N_A, N_B, \ldots$	zero-mean additive noise in A, B,...
σ	standard deviation of noise
$\sigma_{N_A}, \sigma_{N_B}$	standard deviation of noise in A, B,...
R	denoised result
C	similarity value based on correlation analysis
C_l^{H}	similarity value in horizontal direction at level l
Cov	covariance
$\mathrm{Cov}_\mathbf{x}$	local covariance around $\mathbf{x}$
Var	variance
$\mathrm{Var}_\mathbf{x}$	local variance around $\mathbf{x}$
$\bar{A}_\mathbf{x}$	local mean of A around $\mathbf{x}$
$\Omega_\mathbf{x}$	local neighborhood around $\mathbf{x}$
η	weighting function for local neighborhoods
$\bar{\eta}_\mathbf{x}$	mean value of weighting function
w	weighting function for detail coefficients
p	parameter of weighting function controlling the strength of denoising
L	linear combination
g_1, g_2	weights
d	direction
τ	threshold
σ_a	estimated standard deviation of noise
σ_b	reference standard deviation of noise
r_Δ	relative error
$\bar{r}_\Delta$	average relative error
σ_{r_Δ}	variance of relative error
s_Δ	average error, normalized on per-pixel basis
G	weighting image
G^{corr}	correlation coefficient based weighting image
G^{sig}	significance weighting image
τ	threshold
$\hat{h}_{\mathrm{lfil}}$	Fourier transformation of linear filter
$\mathrm{MTF}_{\mathrm{afil}}$	MTF of adaptively filtered image
$\mathrm{MTF}_{\mathrm{orig}}$	MTF of original image
$\hat{k}_{\mathrm{mod}}$	modified reconstruction kernel

B.4 Noise Propagation

ρ_{xx} normalized autocorrelation function/ autocorrelation coefficient function
ϕ_{xx} autocorrelation function
ρ^{fan} autocorrelation of noise in fan-beam projections
ρ^{ipol} autocorrelation of noise after rebinning
ρ^{conv} autocorrelation of noise after convolution
δ Kronecker delta-function

B.5 Noise-Adaptive Bilateral Filtering

$v(\theta_i, \mathbf{x})$ variance contribution from projections at angle θ_i to position $\mathbf{x}$
$\theta_{\max}$ angle with largest variance contribution
$\breve{\theta}_{\max}$ direction of strongest correlation
Var_{H} horizontal variance contribution
Var_{V} vertical variance contribution
σ^2 standard deviation of noise in image
$\sigma^2\text{H}$ standard deviation of noise in image in horizontal direction
$\sigma^2\text{V}$ standard deviation of noise in image in vertical direction
$\sigma^2||$ standard deviation of noise in image in direction of strongest correlation
$\sigma^2\perp$ standard deviation of noise in image orthogonal to direction of strongest correlation
f input data
$\tilde{f}$ filtered output data
c domain filter
s range filter
$\Sigma_{\mathbf{x}}$ covariance matrix of Gaussian filter at position $\mathbf{x}$
$\mathbf{R}_{\mathbf{x}}$ rotation matrix
$\mathbf{D}_{\mathbf{x}}$ diagonal matrix
ν_1, ν_2 singular values
q parameter that controls the maximum degree of anisotropy
d parameter that controls the spatial extension of the domain filter
r parameter that controls the strength of noise reduction

List of Figures

List of Tables

Bibliography

[Bonn 02]   S. Bonnet, F. Peyrin, F. Turiman, and R. Prost. "Multiresolution Reconstruction in Fan-Beam Tomography". *IEEE Transactions on Image Processing*, Vol. 11, No. 3, pp. 169–176, March 2002.

[Bors 06]   A. Borsdorf, R. Raupach, and J. Hornegger. " Wavelet based Noise Reduction by Identification of Correlation ". In: K. Franke, K. Müller, B. Nickolay, and R. Schäfer, Eds., *Pattern Recognition (DAGM 2006), Lecture Notes in Computer Science* , pp. 21–30, Springer, Berlin, 2006.

[Bors 07a]   A. Borsdorf, R. Raupach, and J. Hornegger. "Separate CT-Reconstruction for Orientation and Position Adaptive Wavelet Denoising". In: A. Horsch, T. M. Deserno, H. Handels, H.-P. Meinzer, and T. Tolxdoff, Eds., *Bildverarbeitung für die Medizin 2007*, pp. 232–236, Berlin, 2007.

[Bors 07b]   A. Borsdorf, R. Raupach, and J. Hornegger. "Separate CT-Reconstruction for 3D Wavelet Based Noise Reduction Using Correlation Analysis". In: B. Yu, Ed., *IEEE NSS/MIC Conference Record*, pp. 2633–2638, 2007.

[Bors 08a]   A. Borsdorf, S. Kappler, R. Raupach, and J. Hornegger. "Analytic Noise Propagation in Indirect Fan-Beam FBP Reconstruction". In: E. 2008, Ed., *Proceedings of the 30th Annual International IEEE EMBC Conference*, pp. 2701–2704, 2008.

[Bors 08b]   A. Borsdorf, S. Kappler, R. Raupach, and J. Hornegger. "Analytic Noise Propagation for Anisotriopic Denoising of CT Images". In: P. Sellin, Ed., *2008 IEEE Nuclear Science Symposium Conference Record*, pp. 5335–5338, 2008.

[Bors 08c]   A. Borsdorf, R. Raupach, T. Flohr, and J. Hornegger. "Wavelet based Noise Reduction in CT-Images Using Correlation Analysis". *IEEE Transactions on Medical Imaging*, Vol. 27, No. 12, pp. 1685–1703, 2008.

[Bors 08d]   A. Borsdorf, R. Raupach, and J. Hornegger. "Multiple CT-reconstructions for locally adaptive anisotropic wavelet denoising". *International Journal of Computer Assisted Radiology and Surgery*, Vol. 2, No. 5, pp. 255–264, March 2008.

[Bors 09]   A. Borsdorf, S. Kappler, R. Raupach, F. Noo, and J. Hornegger. "Local Orientation-Dependent Noise Propagation for Anisotropic Denoising of CT-Images". In: *2008 IEEE Nuclear Science Symposium Conference Record*, p. , 2009.

[Bron 00]   I. Bronstein, K. Semendjajew, M. G., and H. Mühlig. *Taschenbuch der Mathematik*. Verlag Harri Deutsch, 5 Ed., August 2000.

[Brud 01]   H. Bruder, T. Flohr, O. Sembritzki, and K. Stierstorfer. "Adaptive filtering of projection data acquired by medical diagnostic device involves adding filtered acquired data to acquired data, determining quantitative ratio of filtered and acquired data". 2001. patent DE1043484.

[Brud 06]   H. Bruder, K. Stierstorfer, C. McCullough, R. Raupach, M. Petersilka, M. Grasruck, C. Suess, B. Ohnesorge, and T. Flohr. "Design considerations in cardiac CT". In: M. Flynn and J. Hsieh, Eds., *Medical Imaging 2006: Physics of Medical Imaging. Proceedings of the SPIE* , pp. 151–163, March 2006.

[Buzu 04]   T. Buzug. *Einführung in die Computertomographie*. Springer-Verlag, Berlin Heidelberg, 2004.

[Catt 92]   F. Catte, P.-L. Lions, J.-M. Morel, and T. Coll. "Image Selective Smoothing and Edge-Detection by Nonlinear Diffusion". *SIAM Journal on Numerical Analysis*, Vol. 29, No. 1, pp. 182–193, 1992.

[Chew 78]   E. Chew, G. Weiss, R. Brooks, and G. Chiro. "Effect of CT noise on detectability of test objects". *American Journal of Roentgenology*, Vol. 131, No. 4, pp. 681–685, 1978.

[Coif 95]   R. R. Coifman and D. L. Donoho. "Translation-Invariant De-Noising". In: *Lecture Notes in Statistics: Wavelets and Statistics*, pp. 125–150, 1995.

[Cunn 92]   I. A. Cunningham and B. K. Reid. "Signal and noise in modulation transfer function determinations using the slit, wire, and edge techniques". *Medical Physics*, Vol. 19, No. 4, pp. 1037–1044, July 1992.

[Daub 92]   I. Daubechies. *Ten Lectures on Wavelets*. Society for Industrial and Applied Mathematics, Philadelphia, 1992.

[Dela 95]   A. Delaney and Y. Bresler. "Multiresolution Tomographic Reconstruction Using Wavelets". *IEEE Transactions on Image Processing*, Vol. 4, No. 6, pp. 799–813, June 1995.

[Demi 01]   O. Demirkaya. "Reduction of noise and image artifacts in computed tomography by nonlinear filtration of projection images". In: M. Sonka and K. M. Hanson, Eds., *Proc. SPIE Vol. 4322, p. 917-923, Medical Imaging 2001: Image Processing*, pp. 917–923, July 2001.

[Denn 09]   F. Dennerlein. *Image Reconstruction from Fan-Beam and Cone-Beam Projections*. PhD thesis, Friedrich-Alexander-University Erlangen-Nuremberg, 2009.

[Dono 94]   D. L. Donoho and I. M. Johnstone. "Ideal spatial adaptation by wavelet shrinkage". *Biometrika*, Vol. 81, No. 3, pp. 425–455, 1994.

[Elba 03]   I. Elbakri and J. Fessler. "Efficient and accurate likelihood for iterative image reconstruction in x-ray computed tomography". In: M. Sonka and J. Fitzpatrick, Eds., *Medical Imaging 2003: Image Processing. Proceedings of the SPIE.*, pp. 1839–1850, May 2003.

[Fagh 02]   F. Faghih and M. Smith. "Combining Spatial and Scale-Space Techniques for Edge Detection to Provide a Spatially Adaptive Wavelet-Based Noise Filtering Algorithm". *IEEE Transactions on Image Processing*, Vol. 11, No. 9, pp. 1062–1071, September 2002.

[Fawc 06]   T. Fawcett. "An introduction to ROC analysis". *Pattern Recogn. Lett.*, Vol. 27, No. 8, pp. 861–874, 2006.

[Fess 97]   J. Fessler, E. Ficaro, N. Clinthorne, and K. Lange. "Grouped-coordinate ascent algorithms for penalized-likelihoodtransmission image reconstruction". *IEEE Trans Med Imaging*, Vol. 16, No. 2, pp. 166–175, April 1997.

[Getr 05]   P. Getreuer. "Filter Coefficients to Popular Wavelets". 2005.

[Giro 01]   B. Girod, R. Rabenstein, and S. A. *Signals and Systems*. Wiley, May 2001.

[Gres 00]   H. Gress, H. Wolf, U. Baum, M. Lell, M. Pirkl, W. Kalender, and W. Bautz. "Dose Reduction in Computed Tomography by Attenuation Based On-Line Modulation of Tube Current: Evaluation of Six Anatomical Regions". *European Radiology*, Vol. 10, No. 2, pp. 391–394, 2000.

[Gres 02]   H. Gress, H. Wolf, C. Suess, J. Lutze, W. Kalender, and W. Bautz. "Automatic Exposure Control to Reduce Dose in Subsecond Multislice Spiral CT: Phantom Measurements and Clinical Results". *Radiology*, Vol. 225, p. 593, 2002.

[Hopp 09]   S. Hoppe. *Accurate Cone-Beam Image Reconstruction in C-Arm Computed Tomography*. PhD thesis, Friedrich-Alexander-University Erlangen-Nuremberg, 2009.

[Hsie 98]   J. Hsieh. "Adaptive streak artifact reduction in computed tomography resulting from excessive x-ray photon noise". *Medical Physics*, Vol. 25, No. 11, pp. 2139–2147, November 1998.

[Hubb 97]   B. B. Hubbard. *Wavelets: Die Mathematik der kleinen Wellen*. Birkhäuser Verlag, Basel, Switzerland, 1997.

[Judy 76]   P. Judy. "The line spread function and modulation transfer function of a computed tomographic scanner". *Medical Physics*, Vol. 3, No. 4, pp. 233–236, 1976.

[Kach 01]   M. Kachelrieß, O. Watzke, and W. A. Kalender. "Generalized multi-dimensional adaptive filtering for conventional and spiral single-slice, multi-slice, and cone-beam CT". *Medical Physics*, Vol. 28, No. 4, pp. 475–490, April 2001.

[Kak 01]   A. Kak and M. Slanely. *Principles of Computerized Tomographic Imaging*. Society for Industrial and Applied Mathematics, July 2001. http://www.slaney.org/pct/pct-toc.html.

[Kale 00]   W. A. Kalender. *Computed Tomography*. Publicis Corporate Publishing, Erlangen, 2000.

[Kale 99]   W. A. Kalender, H. Wolf, C. Suess, M. Gies, and W. Bautz. "Dose Reduction in CT by On-Line Tube Current Control: Principles and Validation on Phantoms and Cadavers". *European Radiology*, Vol. 9, No. 2, pp. 323–328, 1999.

[Kalr 05]   M. K. Kalra, S. M. R. Rizzo, and R. A. Novelline. "Reducing Radiation Dose in Emergency Computed Tomography with Automatic Exposure Control Techniques". *Emergency Radiology*, Vol. 11, No. 5, pp. 267–274, 2005.

[Kats 02]   A. Katsevich. "Analysis of an exact inversion algorithm for spiral cone-beam CT". *Physics in Medicine and Biology*, Vol. 47, No. 15, pp. 2583–2597, July 2002.

[Kunz 07]   H. Kunze. *Iterative Rekonstruktion in der Medizinischen Bildverarbeitung*. PhD thesis, Friedrich-Alexander-University Erlangen-Nuremberg, Juli 2007.

[La R 06]   P. La Rivière, J. Bian, and P. Vargas. "Penalized-likelihood sinogram restora-
            tion for computed tomography.". *IEEE Trans Med Imaging*, Vol. 25, No. 8,
            pp. 1022–1036, 2006.

[Lang 95]   K. Lange and J. Fessler. "Globally convergent algorithms for maximum a pos-
            teriori transmission tomography". *IEEE Transactions on Image Processing*,
            Vol. 4, No. 10, pp. 1430–1438, 1995.

[Li 04]   T. Li, X. Li, J. Wang, J. Wen, H. Lu, J. Hsieh, and Z. Liang. "Nonlinear
            sinogram smoothing for low-dose X-ray CT". *IEEE Transactions on Nuclear
            Science*, Vol. 51, No. 5, pp. 2505–2512, October 2004.

[Li 07]   B. Li, G. Avinash, and J. Hsieh. "Resolution and noise-tradeoff analysis for
            volumetric CT". *Medical Physics*, Vol. 34, No. 10, pp. 3732–3738, October
            2007.

[Lu 03]   H. Lu, X. Li, L. Li, D. Chen, Y. Xing, J. Hsieh, and Z. Liang. "Adaptive
            noise reduction toward low-dose computed tomography". In: M. J. Yaffe and
            L. E. Antonuk, Eds., *Medical Imaging 2003: Physics of Medical Imaging.*,
            pp. 759–766, June 2003.

[Mall 89]   S. G. Mallat. "A Theory for Multiresolution Signal Decomposition: The
            Wavelet Representation". *IEEE Transactions on Pattern Analysis and Mas-
            chine Intelligence*, Vol. 11, No. 7, pp. 674–693, 1989.

[Mall 92]   S. Mallat and S. Zhong. "Characterization of signals from multiscale edges".
            In: *IEEE Transactions on Pattern Analysis and Machine Intelligence*, pp. 710–
            732, July 1992.

[Mall 99]   S. Mallat. *A Wavelet Tour of Signal Processing*. Academic Press, 2 Ed., 1999.

[Maye 07]   M. Mayer, A. Borsdorf, H. Köstler, J. Hornegger, and U. Rüde. "Nonlinear
            Diffusion vs. Wavelet Based Noise Reduction in CT Using Correlation Analy-
            sis". In: *Vision, Modelling, and Visualisation 2007*, pp. 223–232, Saarbrücken,
            2007.

[McCo 06]   C. McCollough, M. Bruesewitz, and J. Kofler. "CT Dose Reduction and Dose
            Management Tools: Overview of Available Options". *RadioGraphics*, Vol. 26,
            No. 2, pp. 503–512, 2006.

[Meye 93]   Y. Meyer. *Wavelets Algorithms & Applications*. Society for Industrial and
            Applied Mathematics, Philadelphia, 1993.

[Naso 95]   G. P. Nason and B. W. Silverman. "The Stationary Wavelet Transform and
            some Statistical Applications". In: *Lecture Notes in Statistics: Wavelets and
            Statistics*, pp. 281–300, 1995.

[Natt 86]   F. Natterer. *The Mathematics of Computerized Tomography*. Wiley and B.G.
            Teubner, Stuttgart, 1986.

[Niem 83]   H. Niemann. *Klassifikation von Mustern*. Springer, Heidelberg, 1983.

[Noo 03]   F. Noo, J. Pack, and D. Heuscher. "Exact helical reconstruction using native
            cone-beam geometries". *Physics in Medicine and Biology*, Vol. 48, No. 23,
            pp. 3787–3818, November 2003.

[Noo 08]   F. Noo. "3D reconstruction techniques in medical imaging". August 2008.
            Lecture notes.

[Oppe 06]   A. Oppelt, Ed. *Imaging Systems for Medical Diagnostics*. Publicis Corporate Publishing, Erlangen, 2 Ed., February 2006.

[Oppe 96]   A. V. Oppenheim, A. S. Willsky, and S. H. Nawab. *Signals and Systems*. Prentice Hall, August 1996.

[Pan 03]   X. Pan and L. Yu. "Image Reconstruction with Shift-Variant Filtration and Its Implication for Noise and Resolution Properties in Fan-beam Computed Tomography". *Med. Phys.*, Vol. 30, No. 4, pp. 590–600, April 2003.

[Pan 99]   X. Pan. "Optimal Noise Control in and Fast Reconstruction of Fan-Beam Computed Tomography Image". *Med. Phys.*, Vol. 26, No. 5, pp. 689–697, May 1999.

[Pizu 03]   A. Pizurica, W. Philips, I. Lemahieu, and M. Acheroy. "A Versatile Wavelet Domain Noise Filtration Technique for Medical Imaging". *IEEE Transactions on Image Processing*, Vol. 22, No. 3, pp. 1062–1071, March 2003.

[Rust 02]   G.-F. Rust, V. Aurich, and M. Reiser. "Noise/dose reduction and image improvements in screening virtual colonoscopy with tube currents of 20 mAs with nonlinear Gaussian filter chains". In: A. V. Clough and C.-T. Chen, Eds., *Proc. SPIE Vol. 4683, p. 186-197, Medical Imaging 2002: Physiology and Function from Multidimensional Images, Anne V. Clough; Chin-Tu Chen; Eds.*, pp. 186–197, April 2002.

[Ruth 76]   R. Rutherford, B. Pullan, and I. Isherwoord. "Measurement of effective atomic number and electron density using an EMI scanner". *Neuroradiology*, Vol. 11, No. 1, pp. 15–21, 1976.

[Star 02]   J. Starck, E. Candès, and D. Donoho. "The Curvelet Transform for Image Denoising". *IEEE Transactions on Image Processing*, Vol. 11, No. 6, pp. 670–684, June 2002.

[Stie 02]   K. Stierstorfer, T. Flohr, and H. Bruder. "Segmented multiple plane reconstruction: A novel approximate reconstruction scheme for multi-slice spiral CT". *Physics in Medicine and Biology*, Vol. 47, No. 15, pp. 2571–2581, August 2002.

[Stie 04]   K. Stierstorfer, A. Rauscher, J. Boese, H. Bruder, S. Schaller, and T. Flohr. "Weighted FBP - a simple approximate 3DFBP algorithm for multislice spiral CT with good dose usage for arbitrary pitch". *Physics in Medicine and Biology*, Vol. 49, No. 11, pp. 2209–2218, June 2004.

[Stra 96]   G. Strang and T. Nguyen. *Wavelets and Filter Banks*. Wellesley- Cambridge Press, 1996.

[Sues 02]   C. Suess and X. Y. Chen. "Dose Optimization in Pediatric CT: Current Technology and Future Innovations". *Pediatric Radiology*, Vol. 32, No. 10, pp. 729–734, 2002.

[Sunn 07]   J. Sunnegardh. *Combining Analytical and Iterative Reconstruction in Helical Cone-Beam CT*. PhD thesis, Linköping University, Juli 2007.

[Tisc 05]   O. Tischenko, C. Hoeschen, and E. Buhr. "An artifact-free structure-saving noise reduction using the correlation between two images for threshold determination in the wavelet domain". In: J. M. Fitzpatrick and J. M. Reinhardt, Eds., *Medical Imaging 2005: Image Processing. Proceedings of the SPIE.*, pp. 1066–1075, April 2005.

[Toma 98]   C. Tomasi and R. Manduchi. "Bilateral Filtering for Gray and Color Images". In: *IEEE International Conference on Computer Vision*, pp. 836–846, Bombay, India, 1998. http://www.cse.ucsc.edu/˜manduchi/Papers/ICCV98.pdf.

[Umwe 08]   "Umweltradioaktivität und Strahlenbelastung im Jahr 2007". Bundesministerium für Umwelt, Naturschutz und Reaktorsicherheit, December 2008. www.bfs.de/de/bfs/druck/uus/pb_archiv.html.

[Vale 04]   C. Valens.   "A Really Friendly Guide to Wavelets".   2004. http://perso.wanadoo.fr/polyvalens/clemens/wavelets/wavelets.html.

[Vest 98]   H. Vestner. "Formeln zum Rauschen in der CT". Technischer Bericht, Siemens Medical Solutions, Forchheim, Juli 1998.

[Wang 05]   J. Wang, H. Lu, T. Li, and Z. Liang. "An alternative solution to the nonuniform noise propagation problem in fan-beam FBP image reconstruction". *Med. Phys.*, Vol. 32, No. 11, pp. 3389–3394, November 2005.

[Wave 06]   *Wavelet   Toolbox.*   Mathworks   Inc.,   2006. http://www.mathworks.com/products/wavelet/.

[Weis]   E. Weisstein.   "Variance".   From MathWorld–A Wolfram Web Resource, http://mathworld.wolfram.com/Variance.html, accessed online October 2009.

[Wick 94]   M. Wickerhauser. *Adapted Wavelet Analysis from Theory to Software.* AK Peters, 1994.

[Wund 08]   A. Wunderlich and F. Noo. "Image covariance and lesion detectability in direct fan-beam x-ray computed tomography". *Phys. Med. Biol.*, Vol. 53, No. 10, pp. 2471–2493, May 2008.

[Xu 94]   Y. Xu, J. B. Weaver, D. M. Healy, and J. Lu. "Wavelet Transform Domain Filters: A Spatially Selective Noise Filtration Technique". *IEEE Transactions on Image Processing*, Vol. 3, No. 6, pp. 747–758, July 1994.